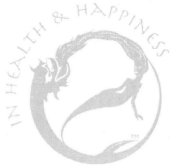

# Welcome to the Prenatal Health and Happiness Program

**Warning**:

The workouts, nutritional information and other health-related research and activities described in the programs presented by Holli Spicer-Clepper were developed by the author to be used as an adjunct to improved strengthening, conditioning, health and fitness. These programs may not be appropriate for everyone. Individuals who suffer from any disease or are recovering from an injury of any sort should consult their physician regarding the advisability of undertaking any of the activities suggested in these programs. The author has been painstaking in her research and the presentation of the material in these programs. She is neither responsible, nor liable, for any harm or injury resulting from this program or the use of the exercises or exercise devices described herein.

Layout and Design: Joling Lee, Holli Clepper
Cover: Joling Lee
Editors: Ruth Pyszczynski, Kofi Robinson, Cara Lawler, Holli Clepper
Models: Lisa Menuck, Monica Schrader, Holli Clepper

# A Word About Copyright

The information presented in this, or any In Health and Happiness publication, seminar, video, DVD or course is the sole property of the author. Copying this material in any form whatsoever is strictly prohibited without written consent from the copyright holder. If you wish to use any materials, such as lecture or workshop handouts, correspondence course manuals, diagrams and text or concepts developed or taught by Holli Clepper, please use the following guidelines to avoid legal action:

1. If you wish to make significant use of any copyrighted material, e.g. duplicate a page for a client or use an illustration in a presentation, prior written permission must be sought from the author. Request for Permission forms are available from Holli Clepper.

2. Whenever using information gained from any secondary source, always credit the referenced source completely and professionally. In the case of In Health and Happiness source, this means the author, In Health and Happiness and the course material. Paraphrasing without proper referencing is considered plagiarism. Whether intentional or not, this is theft of intellectual property and the plagiarist may be prosecuted under copyright law (depending upon the form and amount of the plagiary). Any type of impersonation of another's ideas is entirely unethical and heavily frowned upon in professional circles.

3. Professional referencing usually takes one of two forms: either the original author is indicated by name in the body of the text and a complete reference is included in the list of source material at the end or a number is inserted in the main text beside the borrowed material, with that number corresponding to the reference in the list of credits. There are many accepted methods of citing works. The following are standard; the author's name; title of book, article, course, video, DVD, etc. Title of journal or magazine (if applicable); publisher or producer (if applicable), date of publication/communication (if oral); page number (if applicable).

4. Any In Health and Happiness materials or concepts may not be sold, published or made part of any program for which a fee is charged without the prior written permission of the author.

# CONTENTS

*"As I held you near my heart, I understood at last, the part of me I never met,*
*you don't remember, but I'll never forget."*
- Na Leo, Song: You Don't Remember.

# Preface

## MY STORY

If I knew then what I know now. When I became pregnant I had many unanswered questions. I decided to write this manual based on all the research I did as a personal trainer, group fitness instructor and as a pregnant woman. Included in this manual is all the information I found that was not readily available through many doctors, midwives or even main stream books. I hope the information proves valuable to you and your clients and makes pregnancy that much more enjoyable.

Don't get pregnant before you're 18. That is all you hear as a teenager. I didn't get pregnant before 18; in fact I started to wonder if I could get pregnant at all. After one miscarriage at 38, I found out I was pregnant 8 days before my 40th birthday. I was elated; it was the best birthday present in the whole world.

### Listeria

A bacterial genus that contains seven species. Named after the English pioneer of sterile surgery Joseph Lister, the genus received its current name in 1940. Listeria species are Gram-positive bacilli. The major human pathogen in the Listeria genus is L. monocytogenes. It is usually the causative agent of the relatively rare bacterial disease, listeriosis, a serious infection caused by eating food contaminated with the bacteria. The disease affects primarily pregnant women, newborns, adults with weakened immune systems, and the elderly[23].

Then the worrying began. Had I drank too much alcohol? Will I get listeria from the pate and feta cheese I ate? Will he be a slow learner because I am a coffee addict? Is my baby OK? Most books out there assured me that I didn't need to worry, but I did need to start focusing on what to do now that I knew I was pregnant.

### Round ligament pain

The round ligaments surround your uterus in your pelvis. As your uterus grows during pregnancy, the ligaments stretch and thicken to accommodate and support it. These changes may occasionally cause pain on one or both sides of your abdomen, typically first noticed during the second trimester.[23]

Then, there is the whole weight gain thing. I remember shopping with my Mom when I was about 8 weeks pregnant and I held up a cute pair of cords and said, "these will be perfect for me as I get bigger, they have such a low waist." Naïve. My Mom laughed to herself thinking "yeah, like the only thing that will get big is your belly." She let me buy them thinking my butt and thighs would stay the same size. Boy was I wrong. As my belly grew, the rest of me stayed relatively the same for a while and then, out of nowhere, my butt expanded and my inner thighs took on a shape I have never witnessed on my frame. Yikes! But of course this will all go away once the baby is born, I'm in shape.

About 4 months into it, I got horrible round ligament pain, which almost feels like you are having contractions. You may feel round ligament pain as a short jabbing sensation or a sharp, stabbing pain if you suddenly change position, such as when you're getting out of bed or out of a chair or when you cough, roll over in bed, or get out of the bathtub. You might also feel it as a dull ache after a particularly active day – when you've been walking a lot or doing some other physical activity. You may feel the pain starting from deep inside your groin, moving upward and outward on either side to the top of your hips. The pain is internal, but if you were to trace it on your skin, it would follow the bikini line on a very high-cut bikini bottom.

# MY STORY (CONT.)

Then, I started experiencing abdominal cramping when exercising. I have been in pretty good shape my whole life, so I thought this was a huge bonus in the pregnancy department. Not when it comes to tight abs. I spent years teaching my TVA (transversus abdominis) to fire when I lifted anything, in any position, now all I wanted to do was shut it down. My little bambino was trying to grow, but my abs were so tight my body was making it hard for him to expand. So, to get rid of the horrible abdominal cramps and round ligament pain, I had to quit weight training. QUIT WEIGHT TRAINING! That is what I live for, that and surfing, which of course I quit in my first trimester. So now what? You hear about women running marathons when they are pregnant, playing volleyball and skiing and everything was all right for them. Why not me? What they don't tell you about, is what you are taking from your precious little baby when you do run marathons and play sports while you're pregnant. Fluids, nutrients, fats and all those vital things that help them grow. This is the time where you begin to learn that you are giving up a part of yourself to bring this precious child into the world and give to them over and over again, whenever they need you.

This pregnancy was so precious to me, I took the advice of my friend and trainer, Janet, and I slowed down. When it took me so long to get pregnant, why would I jeopardize it when it was only 9 months of my life? So I did what my baby needed. I walked, did "serenity" yoga and on occasion, bicep curls. I learned to enjoy walking and of course, my two little Boston Terriers helped a lot. I have always loved yoga, but it took time to surrender to the fact I needed gentle yoga, and Ashtanga was not what my baby or I needed. Life was good.

I practiced all my breathing exercises, built a "vision board" of my ideal birth, (yes I watched "The Secret") and read every book on natural child birth. I was going to do this drug free, natural and fast just like my friend Cara. Long story short, I had every drug you can imagine, ended up with preeclampsia (a fancy name for swelling like a pig and pregnancy induced high blood pressure) and a C-section.

The dreaded C-section. I was told it was necessary because my little darling's heart rate was decreasing every time I had a contraction and the doctor's didn't think he could survive the strong vaginal contractions of the final birthing stage. My mid-wife was there, whom I trusted and she told me I needed the "vaginal by-pass". So of course, I didn't fight it because my baby was in danger. Well, I have read a lot about that too and he was probably OK but who wants to risk it? Again, I had to surrender.

I had my C-section, more drugs and the first 24 hours was a blur. Thank God my husband wouldn't let little Jake out of his sight. We all went home 3 days later and life was crazy, emotional and magical all at the same time. I was sleep deprived the first 4 weeks or so and crying a lot, but I started to adjust and kept telling myself that the hard times soon will pass, I can do this mother thing, no problem. But, nobody told me I would be wearing maternity clothes for the next 4 months. Good thing I didn't give them away.

Now comes getting back into shape. You quickly learn as a new mother to prioritize what must be done once the little one goes to sleep. Exercise is usually last on the list of house chores, work and hygiene. It seems when you finally start to do your living room workout, the little angel wakes up. He likes you plump. And yes breastfeeding does help you lose weight but not in the chest, abs, inner thighs or arms. So you learn to workout with your little angel.

If you are blessed with a little one who likes the baby jogger, get out there and do it. My little guy hated it for the first 3 months, so I was only able to get in a few short walks using the sling. Very anticlimactic for someone who hates walking and loves to sprint and run stairs. Then when I was finally able to workout a little harder, my neck went out along with my SI Joint (sacroiliac joint). With so much relaxin in my system, it was hard to hold a neck adjustment and my core wasn't strong enough to support my back…so, back to walking.

When Jake turned 6 months old, the weight began to come off, my neck started to stabilize a bit and working out became easier. Every single one of us has a very different experience during pregnancy and postpartum. I wrote this manual and *Postpartum Health and Happiness*, to help all pregnant women make nutritional and exercise choices that make their pregnancy more enjoyable and the postpartum experience a happier one. My goal is to provide you with information you may not have come across and some day look back and say "I wish somebody had told me that". Remember though, everyone is different and each experience is different. I wrote about common issues that happened during my pregnancy and those of my clients and friends. So much of what we experienced and information to help us along our pregnancy journey could not be easily found in most books and the internet. The resources I was able to find were available to me because of the knowledge I gained through my studies as a C.H.E.K Practitioner and Metabolic Typing Advisor.

At the end of my pregnancy journey, all that really mattered was that I had a healthy and happy baby. Everything else was secondary. The most touching quote I read after having Jake was from *Mothering Magazine*.

"Now I hold a piece of the vast world in my arms, a small sliver of the ocean and planets, this tiny bundle of perfect cells working in harmony to be tiny fingers, a beating heart, a miracle of breath and dreams…In the middle of the night when I stumble to respond to his cries, I utter low murmuring noises like a mother cow or she-bear. I nudge my baby close, offer a breast, or stroke his cheek. Without thinking, my body responds to the paragraphs of human biology written deep within my muscles and fleshy curves. I give and keep giving, even when the urge to run is greatest." Christine Rosalie, Mothering Magazine, September – October 2007, Primal Love, pg. 39-41.

Life will never be the same, but when you look back you wouldn't want it any other way. I remember people telling me to cherish these times, as it goes so fast. When you are in the moment of your pregnancy, time seems to stand still, and now my little Jake is 5 and I wonder where the time went. Cherish each moment and always remember to take care of you too.

# About the Author

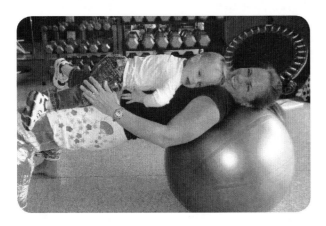

Holli Spicer-Clepper has a B.S. in physical education from Texas A & M, has been a personal trainer, group fitness instructor and educator in the fitness industry for over 23 years. She has taught and trained at a variety of gyms from the YMCA, to Total Woman to the C.H.E.K Performance Studio. She has held Directorial positions in leading health and fitness companies such as the American Council on Exercise from 1991 - 1999 and The C.H.E.K Institute, whom she is still an education consultant for. Holli has taught educational courses for Exercise Etc., The YMCA, and IDEA World, to name a few. She is currently an instructor at the University of California San Diego Extension Program.

Through Holli's unique experience as an educator, personal trainer, C.H.E.K Practitioner and group fitness instructor, she has developed a keen sense for how the body works and has done in-depth research on functional exercise and holistic nutrition. She has taught prenatal exercise classes as well as trained numerous prenatal and postpartum clients over the years. Holli lives in San Diego California with her son Jake and husband Tim.

## ACKNOWLEDGEMENTS

I would like to thank all my friends and family for their help and support in creating this manual, Karen Francis, Robert Spicer, Cara Lawler, Ivan Lawler, Ruth Pyszczynski, Kofi Robinson, Aisha Robinson, Katie Beroukim, Janet Alexander, Lisa Menuck, Monica Schrader, Tim Clepper, Jake Clepper, Kerryann Conway, Maryann Jones and Joling Lee.

To Trish Kelly for all her support in her amazing "serenity" yoga classes. It taught me to truly surrender and connect to my baby boy.

A very special thank you to Paul Chek and Penny Crozier, who gave me the inspiration and tools to write this manual.

To my wonderful husband for his on going support in this project and my beautiful little boy Jake, who always makes everything in this world more wonderful because he is in it!

*"May the long time sun shine upon you and all love surround you"*

- Celtic Prayer

# Objectives

## At the conclusion of this course you will be able to:

1. Identify 5 common issues pregnant women experience and how to relieve them.

2. Write safe and effective exercise programs for pregnant women.

3. Teach at least 20 yoga poses to help pregnant women through their pregnancy.

4. Learn 3 breathing techniques to help reduce stress for pregnant women.

5. Explain why the Choose My Plate (food guide pyramid) may not be the best diet to follow for your body.

6. Identify 5 basic nutrition secrets for a healthy pregnancy and healthy baby.

7. Identify foods that are harmful to pregnant women and their babies.

# How to Complete this Course as a Correspondence Course Only

To maximize your learning potential, it is recommended that you complete the course in the following manner:

1. Read the manual. The first time through, just absorb the information.

2. Next you should read the exam thoroughly. The purpose is not only to pass the exam, but also to be proficient in applying the techniques. The exam questions will help direct your attention to important concepts and information.

3. Practice all the stretches, exercises and yoga poses you are capable of performing with good form. Repeat this process at least twice - not necessarily on the same day - and if possible, also practice teaching them to a willing friend or family member.

6. Now that you have read the manual and have read the exam, it's time to take the exam. Instructions for completing the exam are found on page 223. The purpose of this correspondence course is not to trick you, but to make sure that you are proficient in the areas of knowledge presented. The exam is designed to direct your attention to the areas of importance.

7. Complete the exam in the manual, page 224-231 and return the exam answer sheet and grading request sheet via mail, e-mail or fax to:

> In Health and Happiness
> Exam Grading
> 1966 Spanish Oak Way
> Vista, CA 92081
> USA
> Fax: (+1) 760.727.8369
> E-mail: holli@inhealthandhappiness.com

# Introduction

There is a lot of information out there on prenatal diet and exercise, yet a lot of this information did not address issues that came up again and again for me and my clients. This course will teach you key principles for exercising and eating when you are pregnant and carry you all the way through birth. *Postpartum Health and Happiness* will expand on breastfeeding, infant development and children's nutrition including exercises and yoga poses to get your body back into shape.

These principles are founded on lifestyle changes that will empower you to be stronger and healthier for life. Whether you are just thinking about getting pregnant, newly pregnant, had a C-section or natural birth, you're a vegan or a meat eater, a professional athlete or couch potato, this course will teach you how to handle all the changes your body may soon see, through optimal nutrition and exercise.

Lastly, everyone is different and needs to address challenges that come up in their pregnancy, day by day and week by week. Several additional resources are cited in the back of this manual. If some of your challenges were not addressed here, please refer to the resource section on page 222, to help guide you to a resource that meets your needs. This manual is not intended to replace the many resources out there, it is simply meant to compliment those resources with a holistic and functional approach.

Entering the world of motherhood, or training a client who is soon to be a mother, is no easy task. I hope this course helps bring to light some information that makes each pregnancy the most enjoyable time of your life.

**Note: This course was written to the lay person with the intention of making it easier to share with your clients.**

# Real issues that may come up in your pregnancy that are not often addressed

There are a great deal of resources out there guiding you week by week through your pregnancy. Two of my favorites were "What to Expect When Your Expecting" by Heidi Murkoff, Arlene Eisenberg and Sandee Hathaway, B.S.N[16], and "Your Pregnancy Week by Week" by Dr. Glade B. Curtis, OB/GYN[10]. As detailed as these books were, they focused on the unfit population and didn't thoroughly address problems such as abdominal cramping due to muscle tightness, round ligament pain, sacroiliac pain (SI) pain and headaches.

## ABDOMINAL CRAMPING

When I became pregnant, I was in great shape and thought I was going to have an easy pregnancy because I was so fit. Wrong! Being fit helped in many ways, but the muscle tightness I had created in my body did not allow room for my baby to grow. After the first trimester, I had to quit weight training to allow my abdominals to relax and make room for my baby. I used yoga to teach my abdominals how to relax. Most books will tell you the opposite and in fact encourage you to keep the "abs" in shape to help support your back. If your abdominals are weak, this may be good for you, but if your core, back and glutes (buttock muscles) are already strong, you may be better off not training your abs during your pregnancy. Bottom line, listen to your body and do what is right for you. A strong set of glutes and a strong back will help alleviate back pain during pregnancy.

## ROUND LIGAMENT PAIN

The other thing that came up for me again and again was round ligament pain. I remember a friend of mine, who just had a baby making fun of me saying "round ligament pain, I have never heard of it, are you sure you're not imagining things." I burst into to tears because it was so real to me, yet so many people had never heard of it. I remember lying on the floor for hours in a fetal position wishing the pain away and being equally scared it was pre term labor. My midwife would calm me down and tell me to just lie in a fetal position and allow the ligament to relax. Round ligament pain can be brought on by long hours of standing or sudden changes of position. Round ligament pain is a sudden stabbing sensation in the groin area which is a result of the stretching of muscle fibers in the round ligament of your uterus, see illustration 1. To reduce round ligament pain you can try the following exercises:

Fetal position - side lying savasana - page 148
Cat/Cow – page 118
Hip extension – page 63
Downward dog - page 133

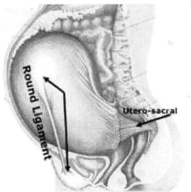

Illustration 1: Round ligament
From: flourishandthriveyoga.blogspot.
com -

## SACROILIAC JOINT PAIN (SI JOINT PAIN)

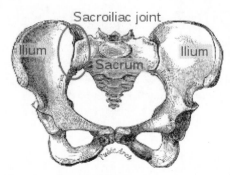

Illustration 2: Sacroiliac Joint

SI Joint pain is frequent during pregnancy for several reasons: Subluxed atlas, weak core, anterior pelvic tilt, relaxed ligaments and weak glutes. There were times when I took a step, it felt like my low back was going to collapse. For me, the issue was primarily an atlas subluxation due to laxed ligaments and previous neck injuries. For each pregnant woman, the cause of SI joint pain will be different and it is important to stabilize this joint to reduce pain and prepare for birth. First, it is important to find out what is driving the SI Joint pain. In illustration 2, you can see where the ilium meets the sacrum. Typically this is a very stiff joint, but during pregnancy this joint becomes more loose as you get ready for labor and delivery of the baby.

It is important to try and stabilize this joint as much as possible through exercises and mobilizations. A compression belt will help stabilize the joint while you exercise or during activities of daily living. A good compression belt can be found at  http://optp.com/Compressor-Belt-Series.aspx.

Seeing a good NUCCA chiropractor also helps a great deal during your pregnancy and you can still get help without x-rays. To find a NUCCA chiropractor go to www.nucca.org (national upper cervical chiropractic association) for a list of NUCCA chiropractors across the world. If for any reason seeing a NUCCA chiropractor is not an option, the following exercises will help stabilize your SI Joint:

Hip extension from floor - page 63
Supine hip extension back on ball – page 64
Sumo squats – page 60
Lower abdominal #1-2 (first trimester and postpartum) – page 96
DonTigny Knee Reach – page 50
Sacroiliac Joint Release with Chair - page 51

## DIASTASIS RECTI

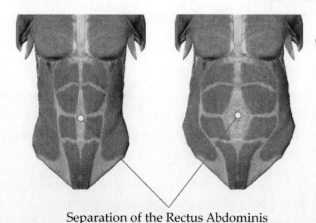

Separation of the Rectus Abdominis
as the abdomen expands

source: visiblebody & core concepts

Illustration 3: Diastasis Recti

Diastasis Recti is the splitting of the abdominal wall, usually caused by a combination of hormonal softening of tissue, the stretching of muscle and sometimes excessive strain occurring in later pregnancy when the muscles are in a lengthened state[18]. This is why it is important to avoid sit ups and jack knife type exercises during your pregnancy. You know you have a significant separation of the abdominal wall if you can fit three or more fingers in the vertical gap (picture on the right). It is important to close this gap, as your abdominals support your back and hold your organs in. See page 94 for the exercise description during pregnancy. A normal gap is when you can only fit 1-2 fingers in the gap. After the baby is born, the same prenatal crunch can be performed where the split has occurred. Please see *Postpartum Health and Happiness* for additional exercises.

## SCIATIC NERVE PAIN

The sciatic nerve runs under your uterus to your legs. The cause of sciatic nerve pain is thought to be associated with pressure on the nerve caused by the developing baby. One way to relieve sciatic nerve pain is to lie on your side, opposite of the pain, side lying savasana, see page 148. Additionally, yoga poses may help relieve pressure on the nerve, see page 112 for a list of poses. Avoid heavy lifting and minimize standing for long periods of time. If you experience pressure while standing, try elevating one foot and resting it on something. Swimming may also ease discomfort.

## Q-ANGLE

Females have a wider pelvis to support child bearing, which creates a larger Q-angle (this is the angle formed by a line drawn from the anterior superior iliac spine through the center of the patella and a line drawn from the center of the patella to the center of the tibial tubercle[24]). An increased Q-angle is often associated with knock knees, pronation, lateral patella tracking, IT band syndrome, chronic knee tracking dysfunctions, varicose veins and Achilles tendon issues. Creating good posture and stability in the pelvis and strength in the glutes, will help decrease a great deal of the issues caused by an increased Q-angle. This is important to begin working on while you pregnant and continued postpartum. Further, once the baby is born, women tend to create a pelvic shift to one side when they balance the baby on their hip for long periods of time. It is important to be mindful of when you do this and try to correct this pattern as often as possible so you do not continue to hang off your connective tissue and ligaments, creating further imbalances in the body. A good overall strength training program will help maintain balance in the body as our body shifts to adapt for the new baby in our lives.

## CONSTIPATION

It is very common for women to become constipated during and after pregnancy. Eating a healthy diet will always help move your bowels, as well as exercise. Be cautious of eating "more fiber" in your diet, as sometimes the foods that contain "more fiber" such as high fiber cereals, oatmeal, prunes etc. can cause constipation. You will learn more about healthy eating in the nutrition chapter. Bottom line, sometimes you will need a safe alternative supplement to get the bowels moving.

I suggest the following resources: **www.herbdoc.com**, Dr. Schultze has an excellent formula called Intestinal #3 that helps move your bowels and may be safe to take during pregnancy. Every pregnancy is different, so please consult your physician before taking this. Sonne's - Herbal Supplement #9a - 100 Tablets which can be found on Luckyvitamin.com, again check with your physician before taking this.

## HEADACHES

For several weeks I was getting severe headaches. In my research I found using a pinch of sea salt in my water, eating at least 3 eggs a day and a dozen shrimp cured my headaches right away. My body was finally getting the nutrients it needed. I only ate the high amount of eggs and shrimp for about a week and the headaches were gone for good.

Our bodies are smart and often let us know when we are lacking in nutrients through pain, discomfort and disease, therefore, it is important to pay attention to what are our body is telling us. See the chapter on nutrition for more information on eating foods high in good fat, vitamin A and vitamin D, see pages 205-206.

# SPLITTING OF THE VAGINAL WALL

Splitting of the vaginal tissue and perineal muscles is quite common and often have varying degrees of tears. Not all tears heal well and additional physical therapy made be needed. A Tens machine has been a very valuable source for several of my clients. Contact your physicial about using a Tens machine if your vaginal muscles are not regaining strength and you have frequent flatulence during the day from the vagina. Below is some great information from Baby Center[6] on vaginal tears.

Is there anything I can do to prevent tearing?
Possibly. Doing perineal massage in your third trimester may help make the skin of your perineum more stretchy and make it less likely that you'll tear or need an episiotomy.

You're also less likely to tear if you have a slow, controlled delivery that allows plenty of time for your perineum to stretch to accommodate your baby. This can mean waiting and fighting the urge to push for a while when the baby's head is crowning, for example. In one study, the use of warm compresses on the perineum during the latter part of the second stage of labor (pushing) was linked to a lower risk of serious tears.

See Postpartum Health and Happiness for more information on recovering from a tear.

## QUIZ #1

1. A sudden stabbing sensation in the groin area can be a result of too much stretch placed on which ligament?

   _____

2. Which hormone can cause the muscles and joints to relax during pregnancy?

   _____

3. The medical name for splitting of the abdominal wall is:

   _____

4. Which nerve does the baby tend to place pressure on during pregnancy?

   _____

5. When the pelvis is tilted _____, it can cause sacroiliac joint pain.

   _____

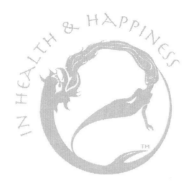

# PRENATAL EXERCISE

# Pregnancy and Exercise

## What you will learn in this section:

- Prenatal exercise guidelines for stretching, strength training, cardiovascular exercise and yoga.
- Common prenatal structural issues that occur and how to alleviate them through stretching, strength training and yoga.
- Several postural exercises to bring the body back to a state of balance.
- Several prenatal exercise routines to help balance the body for a healthy and happy pregnancy.
- Several prenatal yoga sequences to help balance the body and help you to surrender.

## Introduction

It is important to move during your pregnancy. How much will be determined by your previous fitness level, your body's ability to adapt to your pregnancy and your overall physical and mental state. This section was developed to give you the tools you need to stay healthy during your pregnancy, while calming your mind and body as you get ready for the birthing process. Maintaining good posture during your pregnancy will be essential to allowing your body to adapt well to your pregnancy and reduce the amount of pain that is often brought on by postural dysfunctions.

Very specific guidelines and cues are given for each exercise, but remember to always consult your physician before starting or continuing an exercise program during pregnancy.

# Exercise Guidelines

## PROTECTING YOUR BODY DURING AND AFTER PREGNANCY

During pregnancy, females become very rounded in their upper backs, their pelvis falls forward into an anterior pelvic tilt and their knees start to come together. As gravity takes over and the weight of the baby increases, it becomes harder and harder to maintain good posture. Therefore, it is important to be mindful of your posture in everything that you do, in order to maintain a healthy and happy body. Learn to lift with your legs and to sit and stand tall as often as possible. When reaching in and out the car for groceries, or performing a similar movement pattern, always find a way to perform these movements using your large butt muscles, and/or drawing your belly button in and protecting your back.

## INCONTINENCE

Incontinence is very common among females before, during and after pregnancy. Having a strong inner core is essential to preventing incontinence, especially following a c-section. The transversus abdominis, which lies behind the belly button, is only one muscle in the inner-unit of the core that helps stabilize the back and prevent incontinence. The other muscles of the inner-unit, which are on the same neurological loop as the transversus abdominis are the multifidus, pelvic floor, diaphragm and posterior fibers of the internal obliques. If any of these muscles are not functioning properly, incontinence may occur. Therefore, exercises such as lower abdominal #1, tummy vacuums, horse stance and kegels are very important not only for protecting the back, but also for preventing incontinence.

## CORE EXERCISES DURING PREGNANCY

Every woman is different during their pregnancy, therefore each woman should rely on her body to tell her if an exercise is helping her or hurting her. It is important to maintain a strong core throughout your pregnancy, but not to the extent you would when you are trying to get a "wash board stomach". Your baby needs room to grow and your abdominals may cramp if you over work them and create too much tightness in the abdominal wall. When doing any core exercises during your pregnancy, back off if your abdominals start to cramp and let the abdominals relax.

## SACROILIAC JOINT PAIN (SI JOINT) AND LOW BACK PAIN

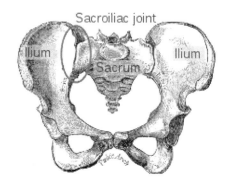

As discussed on page 18, a woman will frequently experience SI Joint pain in the lower back region during pregnancy. The weight of the baby will start to pull the mother into anterior pelvic tilt creating a very unstable SI Joint. As the SI joint becomes unstable, pain and instability are often felt in the low back. Performing sumo squats as seen on page 60 and DonTigny knee reaches on page 50, can help stabilize the SI Joint and provide pain relief. It is important for all females to keep their gluteus maximus (buttocks) strong to support the low back during pregnancy and postpartum.

Illustration 4: Sacroiliac Joint

# THE HORMONE RELAXIN

According to my research, back pain during pregnancy can be caused by two things: First, as the baby gets larger, the abdominal wall stretches to accommodate the expanding baby, and the extra room needed for this has to come from somewhere. Because the abdominal muscles are stretched far beyond their normal state during pregnancy, they lose their ability to stabilize the spine and maintain good posture, and as a result, the lower back takes on an abnormal amount of weight from the torso, causing an anterior pelvic tilt.

The hormone relaxin is the second explanation for low back pain. During pregnancy, the hormone relaxin is present in 10 times its normal concentration in the female body. Relaxin is good in the sense that it relaxes the joints in the pelvis so the baby has room to pass through the birth canal. Unfortunately, relaxin also causes abnormal motion in many other joints of the body, causing inflammation and pain. Therefore, creating strength and stability in the body is very important.[2]

# THORACIC EXTENSION

It is extremely important that as a mother's breasts and belly get larger, they are able to maintain their thoracic extensor strength, (the place between your shoulder blades). As the thoracic spine begins to round, the head comes forward and places a great deal of stress on the cervical spine, mid and low back. If this is not corrected, shoulder and neck pain will also develop over time, as the thoracic spine must be able to go into extension during any arm raise or the shoulder will take the brunt of the lift.

The foam roller mobilization on page 40, is an excellent tool for keeping the thoracic spine from becoming too rounded, as is the bent over row on page 70, or any pulling exercise that is easy for the mother to perform.

# YOUR NECK AND FEEDING YOUR BABY

Looking at your baby and making eye contact during breast or bottle feeding is extremely important to your relationship with your child and almost impossible not to do. However, this can be a very stressful position for your neck and causes the neck extensors (muscles in the back of the neck) to become weak. It is important to maintain your neck strength as you get ready for breastfeeding. Some great exercises are the wall lean and horse stance exercises with a dowel rod, found on pages 33-34, in the postural section.

# WRIST STRENGTH

During the first 2 years of a child's life, mothers tend to hold them in positions that not only compromise the back, but also the wrists. Wrist strength is important to build while a mother is pregnant and continue to build once the baby arrives. Excellent wrist strengthening exercises are push-ups, power webs and simple vertical dumbbell presses. See pages 86-88, for good wrist strength exercises.

# AMERICAN CONGRESS OF OBSTETRICIANS AND GYNECOLOGISTS (ACOG) GUIDELINES

The ACOG guidelines[2] are a good general resource for exercise and pregnancy. According to ACOG, the hormones produced during pregnancy cause the ligaments that support your joints to become relaxed. This makes the joints more mobile and more at risk for injury. The extra weight in the front of your body during pregnancy shifts your center of gravity and places stress on joints and muscles, especially those in the pelvis and lower back. This can make you less stable, cause back pain, and make you more likely to lose your balance and fall, especially in later pregnancy.

The exercises in the prenatal section are designed to address these issues, help decrease pain, while creating stability.

## According to the ACOG guidelines, it is important to stop exercise and call your health care provider if you have any of these symptoms:

- Vaginal bleeding
- Increased shortness of breath
- Chest pain
- Headache
- Muscle weakness
- Calf pain or swelling
- Uterine contractions
- Decreased fetal movement
- Fluid leaking from the vagina

Remember, women have a decrease in available oxygen for aerobic exercise during pregnancy, therefore, they should exercise at a lower intensity during pregnancy, light to moderate exertion. A woman is performing a certain amount of exercise even when at rest, due to the higher oxygen use. It is important to understand your limitations and recognize that although the guidelines are fairly loose on what intensity a woman should exercise at during pregnancy, you must listen to your body and stop exercising if you feel the exercise is too hard and you cannot carry on a conversation.

There are also guidelines stating that if your core temperature exceeds 102°, you will place the baby at risk, because as your core temperature rises, so does that of the baby.

Easy to moderate exercise intensity can help you stay fit, flexible and comfortable while you're pregnant--but you do have to take care to exercise within your new limits as a pregnant woman. It's particularly important to pay attention to your core body temperature and make sure that you don't overheat.

If you do start to feel yourself overheat, take action to cool yourself down quickly. An elevated core body temperature that is 102 degrees Fahrenheit or higher for 10 minutes or longer can mean big problems for baby. A fetus still developing in the first trimester may suffer defects of the neural tube from an overheated mom; a more-developed fetus may suffer dehydration. Immediately stop exercising if you have any trouble breathing, feel nauseous or start to vomit. If you spot any signs of dehydration, your skin gets clammy, you develop a headache or you suddenly feel tired, stop your workout. Also stop exercising if you start to feel weak or dizzy.

Read more:http://www.livestrong.com/article/423024-pregnancy-exercises-core-body-temperature/[4]

Lastly, be sure to drink plenty of water during exercise, as your body is 70% water. You will need plenty of water to keep yourself hydrated and keep the amniotic fluid content high and full of nutrients. Drink water, before, during, and after exercise.

# THINGS TO BE AWARE OF AS YOU EXERCISE DURING PREGNANCY

1.  Always relax the abdominals or lightly draw your belly button in during exercises to protect the back. After the first trimester rely more on your buttocks and back to support your spine and let the belly button relax.

2.  If it hurts, stop the exercise. Exercises are meant to be pain free. Make a note of what hurts and when and report it to your personal trainer or physician.

3.  Always maintain a neutral spine (35 degrees lumbar curve and 35 degrees thoracic curve), see page 27, through out all of your exercises. Always be mindful not to hyperextend your lower back when standing and during exercises. Tucking your tail bone down and lengthening it can help keep your pelvis from falling forward.

4.  Stay present. Focus on the exercise or stretch the entire time. Focus on your breath, your form and how you feel.

5.  Find a time and location to do your exercises where you will not be interrupted.

6.  There has been a great deal of information out there cautioning pregnant women not to exercise lying on their back or perform side lying rotation due to the possibility of supine hypotension (a fall in blood pressure when a pregnant woman is lying on her back causing her to become dizzy and may reduce blood flow to the uterus). According to Elizabeth Noble author of Essential Exercises for the Childbearing Year, very few woman experience supine hypotension during their pregnancy [18]. Consult your physician about performing back lying and spinal rotation exercises, as many of these exercises help relieve back pain and stress placed on the hips.

## Swiss Ball Sizing

Several stretches and exercises in this manual use Swiss balls, so it is important to get the right Swiss ball for your height. You know you have the right size Swiss ball when you sit on a Swiss ball and your thighs are parallel to the floor or slightly higher if you need more curve in your lower back. The rule of thumb for selecting the right Swiss ball for you is:

Under 5"2" - 45cm Swiss ball
5'2" - 5'8" - 55cm Swiss ball
5'9" - 6'2" - 65 cm Swiss ball
6'3" and above - 75 cm Swiss ball

Not all Swiss balls are created equally, so make sure your Swiss ball is anti-burst up to 1,000 pounds. See the equipment reference section on page 219, for places to purchase a quality Swiss ball.

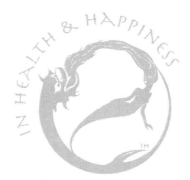

IN HEALTH & HAPPINESS™

# POSTURE

# Posture

Before we begin the exercise section, it is important to note that all of the stretches, exercises and yoga poses in this manual are geared toward bringing the body into a state of good posture, figure 1A. When we are able to maintain good posture, we are better able to handle loads and stresses placed upon our bodies. As we move more into a state of poor posture, figure 1B, our bodies are not able to dissipate the loads and stresses placed upon it and this leads to pain, low back pain, neck pain, knee pain etc.

## What is Good Posture?

From a side view as in figure 1A: Imagine a plumb line hanging about 1 cm forward of the ankle bone. The landmarks the plumb line should bisect are just about midline of the knee, in-line with the greater trochanter of the femur (top of the thigh bone), midway between the back and abdomen as well as midway between the front and back of the chest, through the shoulder joint, and through the lobe of the ear. Ideal curves are 30-35 degrees at cervical, thoracic and lumbar spine, see illustration 5.

From the front or back view the body should be well aligned with the pelvis, shoulders and head sitting level with a straight spine.

## Key Points on Maintaining Good Posture:

- Draw head back so your ear is over your shoulder
- Keep chest lifted - especially as the breasts begin to grow
- Breathe fully and deeply (see breathing exercises on page 32)
- Tuck buttocks under and lightly contract abdominals
- Bend knees slightly when standing

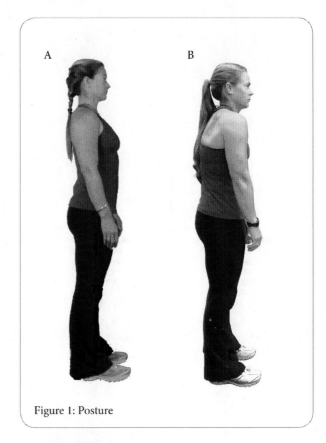

Figure 1: Posture

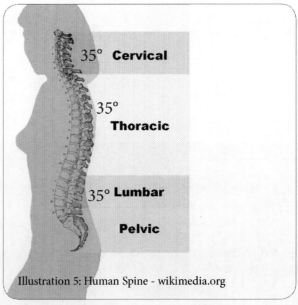

Illustration 5: Human Spine - wikimedia.org

- Distribute weight evenly on both feet

Always be mindful of maintaining good posture throughout each stretch, exercise and yoga pose. If you are starting an exercise program from a place of poor posture, it is essential that you focus on the postural exercises on the following pages to help you restore good posture. Many of the yoga poses will also restore good posture, if done correctly. It is always essential you seek the help of a personal trainer or yoga instructor to ensure that you are doing all of the stretches, exercises and yoga poses properly.

## Poor posture is indicated by the following as seen in figure 2:

- Head coming forward - increases neck pain
- Rounds shoulders - makes it difficult to breath
- Weak, slack muscles in low back
- Forward or anterior pelvic tilt
- Knees hyperextended or locked - strains knees and arches of feet

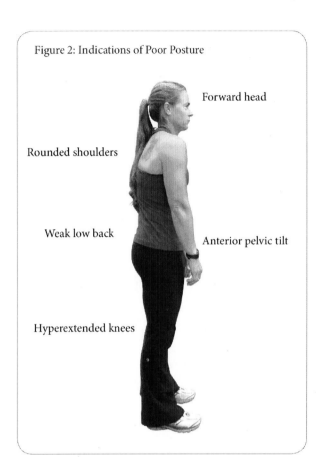

Figure 2: Indications of Poor Posture

Forward head

Rounded shoulders

Weak low back

Anterior pelvic tilt

Hyperextended knees

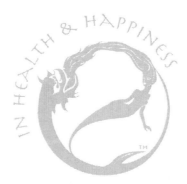

# POSTURAL
# EXERCISES

# BREATHING EXERCISES

## Cues:

1. Stand with your hands on your abdomen as in figure 3A.

2. Breathe into your hands, filling your abdomen first, then your chest.

3. Keep the eyes on the horizon, and exhale from the chest first, then the abdomen.

4. Repeat 5-10 times or until your breath feels comfortable, rhythmic and natural. This may take some time.

## Variations:

1. Move the hands to your sides and breathe into your hands, just like you did when they were on your abdomen, as in figure 3B.

2. Place your hands on your back, as in figure 3C and repeat the breathing exercises as above.

3. Lie on your back with one hand on your chest and one on your abdomen and breathe first into your abdomen, then into your chest, watching your hands rise and then release the breath from the chest, then the abdomen, as in figure 4.

## Variables:

| | |
|---|---|
| Reps: | 1-6 |
| Sets: | 1-3 |
| Tempo: | 6-2-6 or at a slow comfortable pace. |
| Intensity: | Low intensity |
| Rest: | 60-90 sec. |

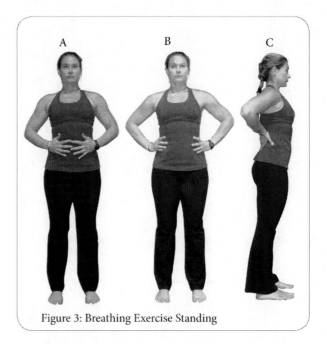

Figure 3: Breathing Exercise Standing

Figure 4: Breathing Exercise Supine

## Precaution:

1. Stop when you feel like you might hyperventilate.

2. If lying on your back causes you to feel dizzy or uncomfortable do not perform exercises on your back.

## Benefits:

1. These exercises teach you how to breathe fully in order to promote healthy posture. When you become a "chest breather," the breath becomes shallow and the head comes forward, creating neck and back pain. In addition, breathing fully allows the body to get the oxygen it needs and helps calm the mind.

# WALL LEAN

## Cues:

1. Stand against a wall with the heels, buttocks, back and head all touching.

2. Move your lower body away from the wall about 6-12 inches keeping the shoulders and head on the wall as in figure 5.

3. Keep the eyes on the horizon, tongue on the roof the mouth and chin parallel to the floor, while pressing your shoulders into the wall.

4. Hold as long as you can and rest for half that time, working up to 3 minutes of total work time.

## Variables:

Reps: 1-6

Sets: 1-3

Tempo: Hold as long as you can and rest 1/2 the time

Intensity: -5 seconds (stop when you can hold for 5 more seconds with good form)

Rest: 60-90 sec.

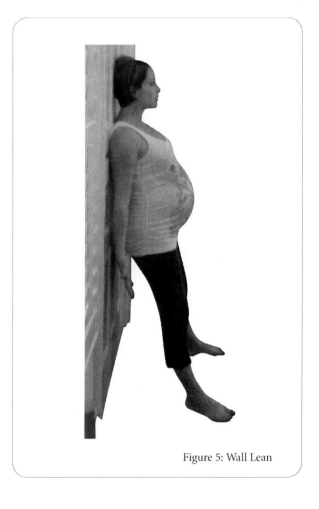

Figure 5: Wall Lean

## Benefits:

1. This exercise teaches your neck and back muscles how to work to hold your body in good posture. In addition, it helps to decrease forward head posture, while working the neck extensors.

# HORSE STANCE

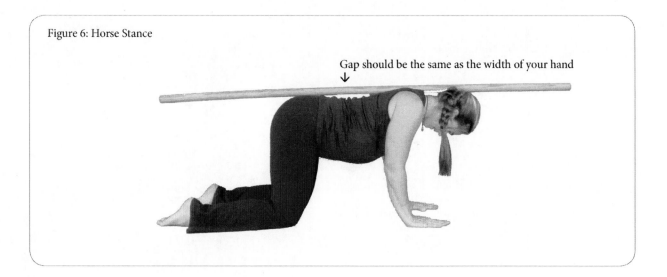

Figure 6: Horse Stance

Gap should be the same as the width of your hand
↓

## Cues:

1. Get on all fours with a stick on your back. Maintaining three points of contact on the stick; head, mid-back and buttocks, figure 6. Maintain neutral spine, drawing the belly button in lightly.

2. Turn the elbows back toward the thighs.

3. Lift the opposite knee and hand off the floor, just high enough for a piece of paper to fit underneath.

4. Hold for 10 seconds and switch sides.

## Modifications:

1. To increase intensity, raise the opposite arm and leg keeping the arm at a 45 degree angle, thumb to the ceiling as in the superwoman exercise on page 72.

## Variables:

Reps:   5-10

Sets:   1-3

Tempo:   10 seconds on 10 seconds off

Rest:   60-90 sec.

## Benefits:

1. This is an excellent exercise to work the small stabilizers and rotators of the spine. In addition, it helps to decrease forward head posture, while working the thoracic and neck extensors.

# CRAWL PATTERN

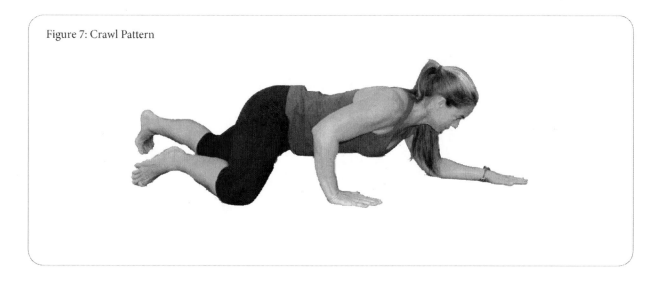

Figure 7: Crawl Pattern

## Cues:

1. Get on all fours and crawl like an infant, alternating sides so that as you reach with your left hand, you are pushing off the right knee as in figure 7.

2. Crawl for 10-20 reps.

## Modifications:

1. This can be done standing, taking your right elbow to the left knee and switching sides each time.

## Variables:

Reps: 10-20

Sets: 1-3

Tempo: slow

Rest: 60-90 sec.

## Benefits:

1. This is an excellent exercise to integrate the left and right sides of the body for people who have poor posture.

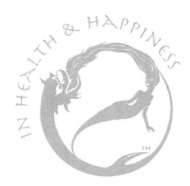

# PRENATAL FLEXIBILITY

# Prenatal Flexibility

## During Pregnancy

Stretching during pregnancy may not be necessary, however, some stretches will feel great to the low back, hamstrings and hips. During pregnancy, yoga poses for short holds and mobilizations will be most beneficial to relax muscles and get the blood pumping through your body. Remember that a hormone called relaxin kicks in during the third trimester, causing the joints to become loose as you get ready for childbirth. Be mindful of how you feel during this time and do not stretch muscles that feel loose or joints that feel unstable. Also be careful with side to side movements, as you may begin to lose the ability to stabilize your body as your hips become looser and looser. See page 24 for more information on relaxin.

# MUSCLE ENERGY EXERCISES AND MOBILIZATIONS

Muscle energy exercises and mobilizations are excellent for actively mobilizing joints and can be used to help with movement restriction. According to Paul Chek[6], in some cases muscle energy exercises and mobilizations are better than static stretching, as the body feels less threatened when it has an active part in the process and allows the joints to move much more freely. If you feel tight and restricted during movement and static stretching does not seem to be helping you, limit yourself to muscle energy exercises and mobilizations on pages 40-42 for a few weeks and see if you notice a difference. Static stretching can cause a guarding response in the body and may actually cause the body to tighten a muscle to protect the joint from being stretched to too great a range of motion.

It is important to only use short stretch times such as 5-10 seconds, muscle energy exercises and mobilizations when preparing the body for exercises. Long, static stretches prior to exercise can actually sedate the muscles being used and does not allow the brain to effectively monitor the length change in the muscle. As a result the brain immediately notices that the information coming from the muscles used to "squat push press" does not match the information stored in the brain as "squat push press". The brain will then try to figure out, mid-exercise, how to modulate the squat to make it match what is stored in the brain, which can lead to injury.

> ## Note:
>
> Foam rollers used in this program are Etha foam rollers and are hypo allergenic. The best size for the mobilizations used in this program is 4 inches in diameter by 3 feet long. These foam rollers can be purchased at www.optp.com.

# STATIC STRETCHES

Static stretches should always be done after exercise, with the goal of improving flexibility and preventing unwanted muscle soreness. The following stretches should be done in the order listed for maximum benefits. When these stretches are done as pre-exercise stretches, which are meant to bring the body back into balance before a workout, the holds will be shorter or done in a contract/relax tempo. Each stretch description will offer the duration of the stretch for pre-exercise goals and post exercise goals, if there is a difference in duration.

To create length in a muscle, the stretches can be done after exercise or before bed, to introduce changes in your posture and alleviate pain. These post-exercise stretches will have longer holds denoted. Stretching should make the body feel better, not worse. If you feel worse after stretching, it is important that you recognize this and then seek the assistance of a qualified C.H.E.K Practitioner or certified Personal Trainer. For a reference on exercise resources, see page 224.

# HORIZONTAL FOAM ROLLER MOBILIZATION

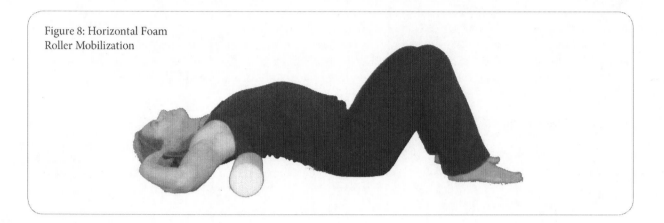

Figure 8: Horizontal Foam
Roller Mobilization

## Cues:

1. First determine where you have a hard time moving in the thoracic spine. This can be done by lifting the arms overhead and feeling where you are "stuck". It is best to have someone observe your spine as your raise your arms, having them observe which vertebrae do not move as you extend.

2. Place a 3"-4" foam roller on this segment with knees bent and arms behind the neck. Be sure to cradle the neck giving it support as in figure 8.

3. Slowly lower the head to the ground and hold for 3 to 5 seconds. If this is difficult for you, simply lower the head and return to the start position, timing the movement with your breath, inhale as you lower, and exhale as you return up.

4. Repeat 3-5 times.

5. Move to the next "stuck" segment and repeat the mobilization.

## Modifications:

1. If this mobilization is hard for you, place a pillow on the floor under your head so your head touches the pillow at a point that is comfortable to hold for 3 - 5 seconds.

2. If this mobilization causes pain, try the vertical foam roller mobilization on page 41.

## Benefits:

1. Opens the thoracic spine. This is a good mobilization to do after breastfeeding or being on your feet all day when you are pregnant.

2. Reduces upper back pain.

3. Opens chest and helps you to breathe better.

## Pre-exercise Variables:

1. Hold 3-5 seconds and come back up, Repeat 3-5 times.

## Post-exercise Variables:

1. Lie back over the foam roller for 30-60 seconds.

# VERTICAL FOAM ROLLER MOBILIZATION

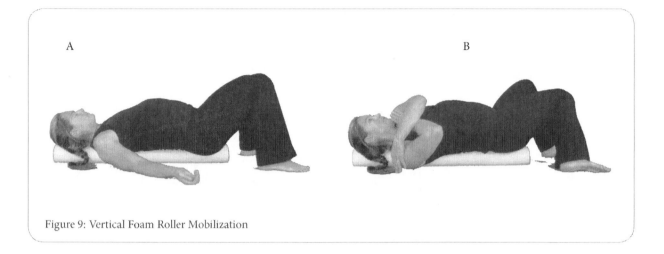

Figure 9: Vertical Foam Roller Mobilization

## Cues:

1. Place a 3"-4" foam roller vertical along your spine so that your head and sacrum are firmly on the foam roller as in figure 9A.

2. Balance on the foam roller with your arms at your side, palms to the ceiling.

3. Hold for 5 minutes and work up to 15 minutes a day.

## Pre-exercise Variables:

1. 5 minutes.

## Post-exercise Variables:

1. Up to 15 minutes.

## Modifications:

1. To increase rotational mobility, you can place your arms across your chest and rotate the upper body one way and the knees the other way, figure 9B. Repeat this process until you feel loose.

## Benefits:

1. Opens the thoracic spine. This is a good mobilization to do after breastfeeding or being on your feet all day when you are pregnant.

2. Reduces upper back pain.

3. Opens chest and helps you to breathe better.

# SWISS BALL PELVIC TILT

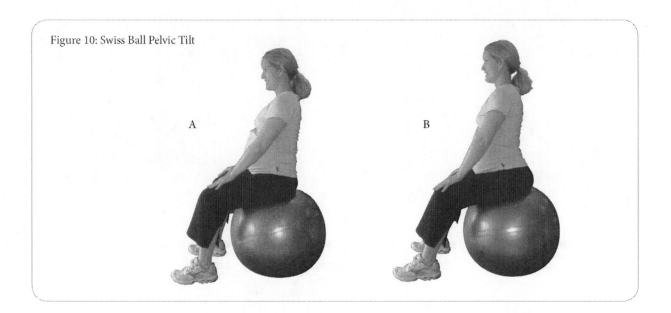

Figure 10: Swiss Ball Pelvic Tilt

A    B

## Cues:

1. Sit on a Swiss ball that is the right size for you (see page 26 for Swiss ball sizing). Your thighs should be parallel to the floor or slightly higher if you have back pain, figure 10A.

2. Plant your feet firmly into the ground and lift your chest. Tuck your pelvis under pulling the ball toward your feet and then tilt your pelvis away from your feet, figure 10B.

3. Continue to do this for 30-60 seconds.

## Modifications:

1. You can draw a figure 8 with the ball, rolling your pelvis right and then left making large circles to open the hips and pelvis.

## Benefits:

1. Opens the hips and pelvis.

2. Reduces lower back pain.

3. Gets the body ready for labor.

4. Can be used as a muscle energy exercise.

## SEATED BACK OPENER

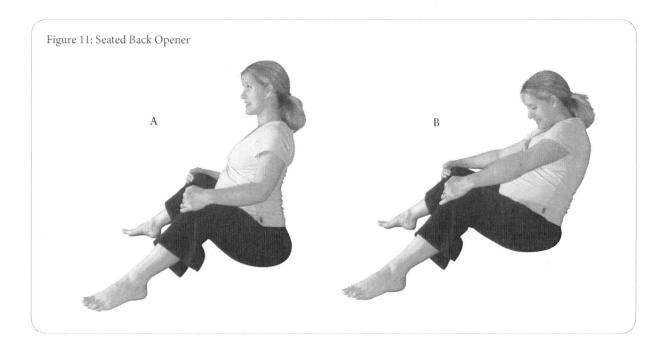

Figure 11: Seated Back Opener

A        B

## Cues:

1. Sit with your knees bent, feet outside your shoulders, grabbing your shins with your hands, pulling your chest up and lengthening your spine, as you inhale, figure 11A. Keep eyes on the horizon.

2. Exhale and round your spine, supporting your back by holding onto your shins, figure 11B.

3. Repeat 5-10 times timed with breath.

## Benefits:

1. Pumps fluid into the pelvic and back area.

2. Stretches low back.

3. Can be used as a muscle energy exercise.

# SWISS BALL HAMSTRING STRETCH

## Cues:

1. Sit on a Swiss ball that is the right size for you. Your thighs should be parallel to the floor or slightly higher if you have back pain.

2. Extend your left leg and place your hands and your right leg.

3. Lift your chest and then tilt your pelvis away from your feet, figure 12. You should feel a significant stretch in the back of the thigh and even in the calf.

3. Hold for 5-10 seconds and switch sides.

## Pre-exercise Variables:

1. 5-10 seconds.

## Post-exercise Variables:

1. Up to 30 seconds.

## Modifications:

1. If you feel unstable on the Swiss ball, this can also be done standing or seated on a chair.

## Benefits:

1. Opens the hamstrings.

2. Reduces lower back pain.

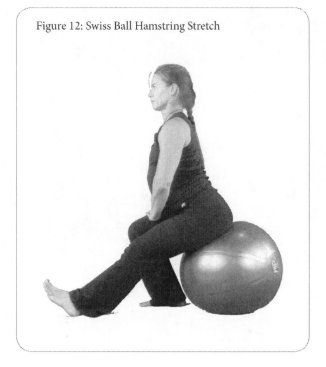

Figure 12: Swiss Ball Hamstring Stretch

# SWISS BALL HIP FLEXOR STRETCH

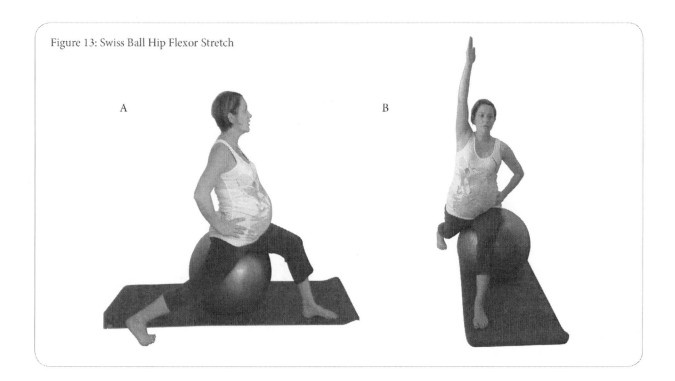

Figure 13: Swiss Ball Hip Flexor Stretch

A

B

## Cues:

1. Sit on the side of a Swiss ball, with one leg forward and one leg back, resting your weight on the Swiss ball, figure 13A.

2. Keep the front knee over the ankle and press the back hip forward creating a stretch in front of the hip on the back leg.

3. Squeeze your buttocks and hold for 5 seconds, relax and exhale as you push the hip on the back leg a little more forward, creating a long stretch in the front of the hip.

4. Hold for 5 seconds and switch sides.

5. Repeat 3-5 times.

## Pre-exercise Variables:

1. 5 seconds, contract, 5 seconds relax or hold for 10 seconds.

## Post-exercise Variables:

1. Hold for 20 - 30 seconds.

## Modifications:

1. Hold a stick or hold onto the wall for balance.

2. If the Swiss ball is hard for you to balance on or you do not have one, you can do the same stretch holding onto a chair.

3. To increase the stretch, lift the arm up and away from the side you are stretching as in figure 13B.

## Benefits:

1. Reduces anterior pelvic tilt, which in turn, reduces back pain.

# GROIN STRETCH

## Cues:

1. Get on knees and place arms in front of you as in figure 14.

2. Push back until you feel a good stretch between the upper thighs.

3. Lightly press the knees into the ground and hold for 5 seconds.

4. Relax and exhale and take the stretch a little deeper and hold for 5 seconds.

## Pre-exercise Variables:

1. 5 seconds contract/5 seconds relax or hold for 10 seconds.

## Post-exercise Variables:

1. Hold for 20 - 30 seconds.

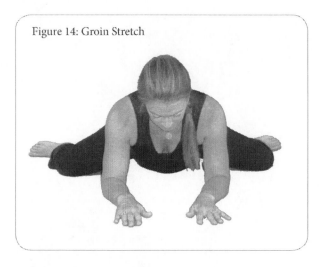

Figure 14: Groin Stretch

## Benefits:

1. Opens up the hips and groin.

# SPINAL ROTATION

## Cues:

1. Lie on back with a block or light ball between your knees, knees bent.

2. Rotate the lower body as far as you can without the opposite shoulder coming off the floor as in figure 15.

3. Hold for 10-20 seconds and switch sides.

## Pre-exercise Variables:

1. Hold for 10 seconds.

## Post-exercise Variables:

1. Hold for 20 - 30 seconds.

## Precautions:

Some pregnant woman may feel discomfort or dizziness when performing a spinal twist. Please consult with a physician before performing this stretch.

## Benefits:

1. Opens up the low back and upper back.

2. Increases spinal rotation needed for picking up your baby.

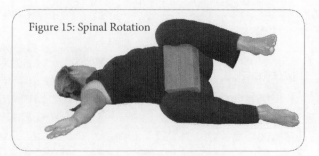

Figure 15: Spinal Rotation

# SWISS BALL RECTUS ABDOMINIS STRETCH

## Cues:

1. Lie over the Swiss ball, with arms extending back, or to the side, figure 16.

2. Rock back and forth for 30-60 seconds to open up the abdominals and stretch the low back.

## Pre-exercise Variables:

1. 30 - 60 seconds rocking.

## Post-exercise Variables:

1. 30 - 60 seconds rocking.

## Benefits:

1. Opens up the chest, low back and abdominal wall.

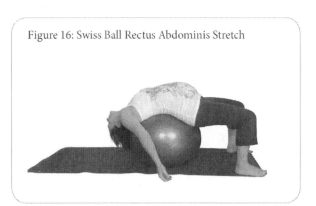

Figure 16: Swiss Ball Rectus Abdominis Stretch

## Precaution:

1. Do not hold longer than 30 seconds during the second and third trimester. If you feel dizzy during the stretch, do not perform this stretch.

# LOW BACK AND GROIN STRETCH

## Cues:

1. Lie on your back and grab the outside edges of your feet with your hands, figure 17.

2. Lengthen your tail bone and gently rock side to side for 5-10 seconds.

## Pre-exercise Variables:

1. Rock 5-10 seconds.

## Post-exercise Variables:

1. Rock 30 - 60 seconds.

## Benefits:

1. Hip, groin and low back opener.

2. Relieves stress and emotions.

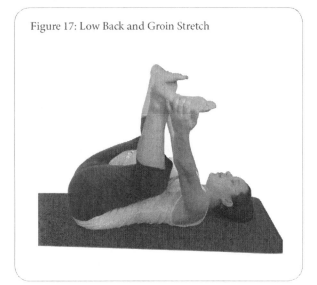

Figure 17: Low Back and Groin Stretch

## Precautions:

1. If lying on your back causes you to feel dizzy or uncomfortable do not perform exercises on your back.

## THREAD THE NEEDLE - UPPER BODY

### Cues:

1. Kneel on the floor. Touch your big toes together and sit on your heels.

2. Reach your left arm under your body and look under your arm with your left ear on the floor.

3. Place your right palm on the floor, finger tips facing you and press into the floor to open the upper back as in figure 18.

4. Hold 5-10 seconds.

5. Switch sides.

### Pre-exercise Variables:

1. Hold for 5-10 seconds.

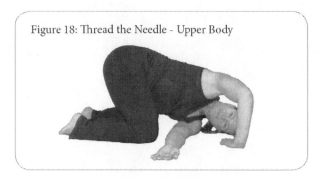

Figure 18: Thread the Needle - Upper Body

### Post-exercise Variables:

1. Hold for 30-60 seconds.

### Benefits:

1. Opens the thoracic spine and shoulders.

## THREAD THE NEEDLE - LOWER BODY

### Cues:

1. Lie on your back with knees bent. Place the right heel on the left upper thigh, figure 19.

2. For a deeper stretch, lift the left foot off the floor and clasp your hands behind your left thigh.

3. Hold this pose for 5 - 10 seconds.

4. Switch sides.

### Pre-exercise Variables:

1. 5 seconds contract/ 5 seconds relax or hold for 5-10 seconds.

### Post-exercise Variables:

1. Hold for 30-60 seconds.

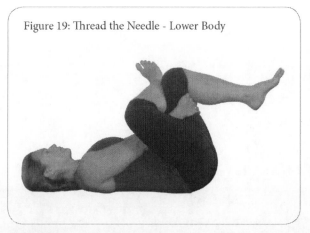

Figure 19: Thread the Needle - Lower Body

### Benefits:

1. Opens the hips.

### Precautions:

1. If lying on your back causes you to feel dizzy or uncomfortable do not perform exercises on your back.

## SWISS BALL PEC MINOR STRETCH

### Cues:

1. Kneeling next to a Swiss ball, place the arm closest to the ball on the ball with the elbow bent at 90°, figure 20.

2. Drop your chest toward the floor until you feel a deep stretch in the chest.

3. Hold this pose for 5 - 10 seconds.

4. Switch sides.

### Pre-exercise Variables:

1. 5 seconds contract/ 5 seconds relax or hold for 5-10 seconds.

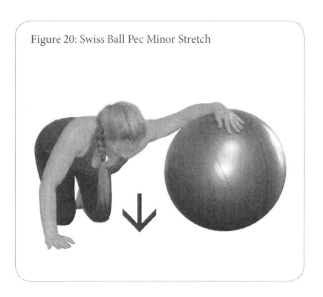

Figure 20: Swiss Ball Pec Minor Stretch

### Post-exercise Variables:

1. Hold for 30-60 seconds.

### Benefits:

1. Opens the chest.

## SWISS BALL PEC MAJOR STRETCH

### Cues:

1. Kneeling next to a Swiss ball, place the hand closest to the ball on the ball as in figure 21.

2. Drop your chest toward the floor until you feel a deep stretch in the chest.

3. Hold this pose for 5 - 10 seconds.

4. Switch sides.

### Pre-exercise Variables:

1. 5 seconds contract/ 5 seconds relax or hold for 5-10 seconds.

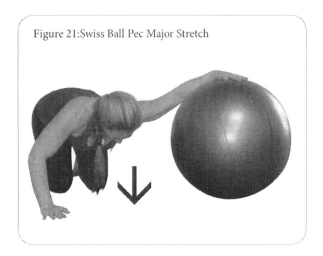

Figure 21:Swiss Ball Pec Major Stretch

### Post-exercise Variables:

1. Hold for 30-60 seconds.

### Benefits:

1. Opens the chest.

# DONTIGNY KNEE REACHES

## Cues:

1. Lie on your back with one leg straight, the other bent, figure 22.

2. Using only the leg that is bent, gently push the knee forward as if a piece of string is attached to the front of your knee and is pulling you forward.

3. Hold for 5 seconds and then relax for 5 seconds and repeat 5 times, switch legs.

4. This is a very gentle push and all movement must be initiated with the knee reach.

## Precautions:

1. If lying on your back causes you to feel dizzy or uncomfortable do not perform exercises on your back.

## Modifications:

1. This can also be done seated or standing as in figure 23A & B. Simply sit or stand tall and pull the knee up and toward the chest without collapsing forward. Hold 5 seconds, switch sides.

## Benefits:

1. Stabilizes the sacroiliac joint, see illustration 6A. The corrections should be done every 2-3 hours throughout the day, for at least three days, to take the tension off of the tight ligaments and give them an opportunity to recover. After that, correct at any sign of recurrence.

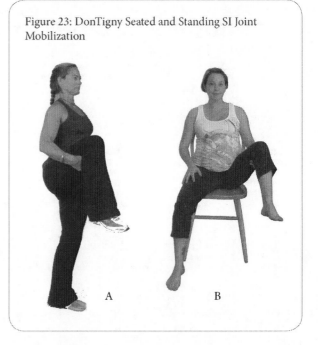

Figure 22: DonTigny Knee Reach Supine

Figure 23: DonTigny Seated and Standing SI Joint Mobilization

A          B

More information on DonTigny can be found at www.thelowback.com

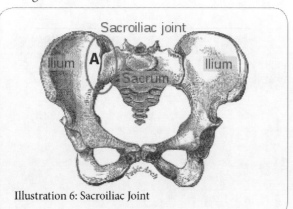

Illustration 6: Sacroiliac Joint

## SACROILIAC JOINT RELEASE WITH CHAIR

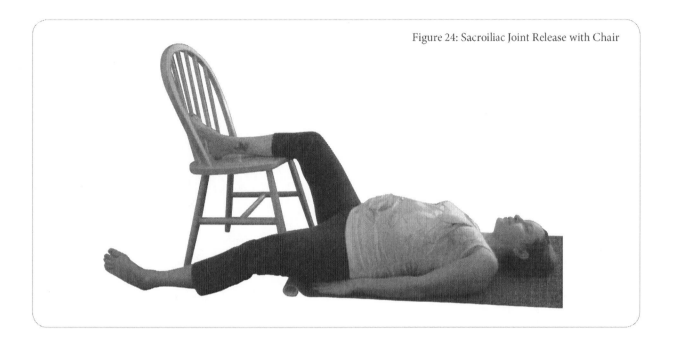

Figure 24: Sacroiliac Joint Release with Chair

## Cues:

1. Lie on your back with one leg straight, and the other leg elevated on a chair, as in figure 24.

2. Hold for 1-5 minutes and switch sides.

## Benefits:

1. Stabilizes the sacroiliac joint. This can be done every 2-3 hours throughout the day, for at least three days, to take the tension off of the tight ligaments and give them an opportunity to recover.

## Precautions:

1. If lying on your back causes you to feel dizzy or uncomfortable do not perform exercises on your back.

## SEATED NECK SIDE FLEXION STRETCH

### Cues:

1. Sit in a comfortable position and grab the chair with your left hand, as in figure 25.

2. Side bend the neck to the right and if you need a greater stretch place the right hand gently on the head and pull.

3. Hold for 5 - 10 seconds and repeat on other side.

### Pre-exercise Variables:

1. 5 seconds contract/ 5 seconds relax or hold for 5-10 seconds.

### Post-exercise Variables:

1. Hold for 30-60 seconds.

### Benefits:

1. Takes tension out of the neck.

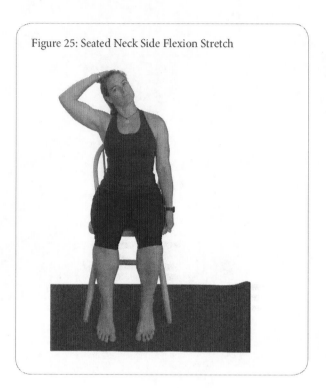

Figure 25: Seated Neck Side Flexion Stretch

## LEVATOR SCAPULAE STRETCH

### Cues:

1. Stand in a comfortable position.

2. Side bend the neck away from the left arm and then look down and toward the left armpit.

3. Hold for 5 - 10 seconds and repeat on other side.

### Pre-exercise Variables:

1. 5 seconds contract/ 5 seconds relax or hold for 5-10 seconds.

### Post-exercise Variables:

1. Hold for 30-60 seconds.

### Benefits:

1. Takes tension out of the neck.

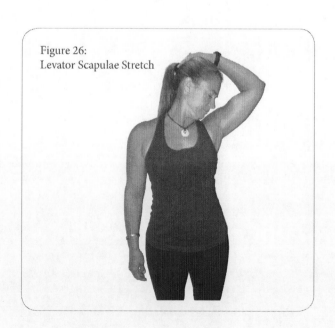

Figure 26:
Levator Scapulae Stretch

# SEATED POSTERIOR NECK STRETCH

## Cues:

1. Sit in a comfortable position and place both hands on the back of your head as in figure 27.

2. Tuck your chin to your chest and take the stretch as far as you comfortably can.

3. Hold for 5 - 10 seconds and repeat on other side.

## Pre-exercise Variables:

1. 5 seconds contract/ 5 seconds relax or hold for 5-10 seconds.

## Post-exercise Variables:

1. Hold for 30-60 seconds.

## Benefits:

1. Takes tension out of the neck.

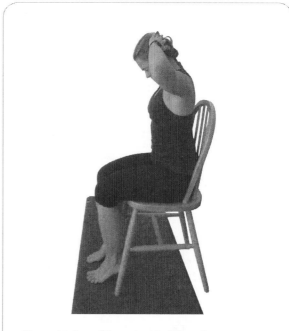

Figure 27: Seated Posterior Neck Stretch

## QUIZ #2

1.   An ideal lumbar curve would be ____ degrees?

   _____

2.   Which stretch helps decrease sacroiliac joint pain?

   _____

3.   Which mobilization helps open the chest and enables you to breathe better?

   _____

4.   Which exercise helps the most with forward head posture?

   _____

5.   Which exercise helps integrate the right and left side of the body?

   _____

## PRE-EXERCISE STRETCH PROGRAM

This sequence helps open up all the muscles that commonly get tight from sitting all day. Please refer to the stretching and mobilization section for more stretches.

| Stretch | Description | Breaths | Notes |
|---|---|---|---|
| | Sit on the side of a Swiss ball with one leg forward and the opposite leg back far enough so you feel a stretch in the front of the thigh. | Hold for 2-5 breaths. | Swiss ball Hip Flexor Stretch page 44 |
| | Sit on a Swiss ball and extend one leg and press the ball back until you feel a stretch in your hamstring (back of the thigh). Place your hands on the bent leg. | Hold for 2-5 breaths. | Swiss Hamstring Stretch page 43 |
| | Get on all fours and place your elbow on a Swiss ball in line with your shoulder. Drop your chest toward the floor until you feel a stretch in the chest. | 2-5 breaths or contract/ relax 5 seconds on 5 seconds off. | Swiss Ball Pec Minor Stretch page 48 |
| | Sit tall and bend your knees grabbing the tops of your shins with your hands. Inhale and pull your chest forward, exhale and round your back. | 5-10 breaths. | Seated Back Opener page 42 |
| | Place a foam roller under your back where you feel "stuck". Keep the knees bent while supporting your neck, let your head come to the floor. | 2-5 breaths. | Horizontal Foam Roller Mobilization page 39 |

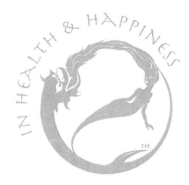

IN HEALTH & HAPPINESS

# STRENGTH
# TRAINING

# STRENGTH TRAINING GUIDELINES

As an athlete, my body has survived many activities, from surfing to rock climbing to scuba diving to Olympic lifting. The hardest thing my body had to endure was pregnancy, breastfeeding, and carrying a baby around all day. I experienced wrist pain, back pain and extreme neck pain that I had never encountered before the first 9 months of my child's life. This strength training section is designed to help get your body ready for pregnancy and all the things to come postpartum. It is a reference tool for aches and pains that will come up and how to relieve them. If you are new to strength training be sure to address any postural issues you may have in the postural chapter on page 27. Of course, always check with your physician before starting any exercise, supplement or nutritional programs.

The following exercises are designed to support the structures of the body during pregnancy, to help create a stable spine and pelvis. Each exercise is listed with a picture and a brief description of how to perform the exercise, along with modifications. Some exercises will include progressions you can use once you can perform the exercise with perfect form for 4-6 weeks.

The following rules apply to all exercises and need to be observed in order to protect your back.

1. Always do needed stretches prior to exercising to bring the body back into a state of balance.

2. Always stop the exercise at the point where you feel that you could only do 2 more repetitions with good form (-2 reps).

3. Please note when the description tells you to draw your belly button in, be sure to relax the belly if this causes cramping.

4. Always stop the exercise if you feel pain and rest for 1-2 minutes. If the pain persists, contact your personal trainer or physician.

# EXERCISE SECTION TERMINOLOGY

## Defining Terms:

Repetitions (reps): Number of times the exercise is to be performed before resting.

Sets: Number of sets of repetitions to be completed in total.

Tempo: The speed at which the exercise is to be performed. For example, a tempo of 2-2-2 means contract for 2, hold for 2 and slowly release for 2.

Intensity: This is the amount of effort you should be using for the entire set. -2 reps means to stop when you feel like you could still perform 2 more repetitions with good form.

Rest: This is the amount of time you should rest in between sets.

Each exercise variable is given as a range because your body can perform differently on a day to day basis. Say you have a rep range of 8-12 and you are feeling particularly tired that day, only perform 8 reps and rest 90 seconds instead of just 60 seconds. If you are feeling strong that day perform 3 sets instead of 2, etc.

At the end of the exercise section are several workout routines you can do, depending on where you are at in your pregnancy and how you are feeling.

## Swiss Ball Sizing:

Several exercises in this section use Swiss balls, so it is important to get the right Swiss ball for your height. You know you have the right size Swiss ball when you sit on a Swiss ball and your thighs are parallel to the floor or slightly higher if you need more curve in your lower back. The rule of thumb when selecting the right Swiss ball for you is:

Under 5'2" - 45 cm Swiss ball
5'2" - 5'8" - 55 cm Swiss ball
5'9" - 6'2" - 65 cm Swiss ball
6'3" and above - 75 cm Swiss ball

Not all Swiss balls are created equally, so make sure your Swiss ball is anti-burst up to 1,000 pounds. See the equipment resource section on page 224 for places to purchase a quality Swiss ball.

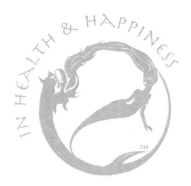

IN HEALTH & HAPPINESS

TM

# LOWER BODY & BALANCE SECTION

# SUMO SQUAT

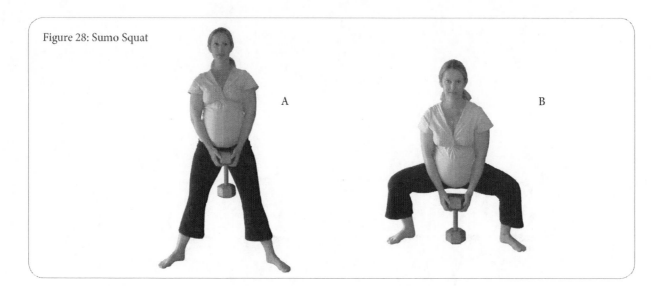

Figure 28: Sumo Squat

A

B

## Cues:

1. Start with feet wider than shoulder width apart and turn the toes out approximately 15 degrees, knee tracking over the second toe as in figure 28A. Hold a dumbbell in your hands and lift your chest.

2. Inhale, belly button in lightly and hold (this helps create a corset effect on the spine, stiffening the spine and protecting it). If you begin to cramp, simply contract your pelvic floor (pretend you are stopping yourself from urinating) and focus on using the buttocks and thighs to protect your back.

3. Bending from the knees, and sitting back as if sitting in a chair, slowly sit into a squat. Keep your chest lifted and a 35 degree curve in the low back, shoulder blade pulled together, as in figure 28B.

4. Go as far as you can while maintaining a 35 degree lumbar curve, keeping your shins vertical (do not let your knee go over your toes). Stop when you feel you are about to lose your curve and feel your back muscles working too hard.

5. As you come up out of the movement, press through your heels and slowly exhale through pursed lips.

## Modifications:

1. If you feel like you are using your low back to perform the exercise, simply shorten your range of motion.

2. If your balance is off, place a Swiss ball on a wall behind as on page 61, to help you maintain your balance and form.

3. This exercise can also be done holding your baby instead of a dumbbell postpartum.

## Variables:

Reps: 8-12

Sets: 1-3

Tempo: 3-1-3

Intensity: -2 reps (stop when you can do 2 more reps with good form)

Rest: 60-90 sec.

## Benefits:

1. This exercise provides excellent lifting mechanics as well as strengthening all the structures that support the pelvis and back. In addition, it helps to stabilize the sacroiliac joint.

# SWISS BALL WALL SQUAT

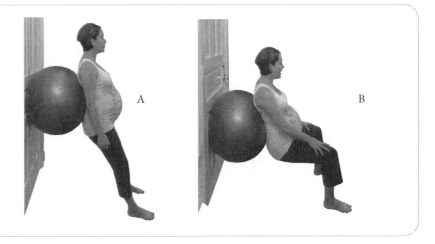

Figure 29: Swiss Ball Wall Squat

A

B

## Cues:

1. Place a Swiss ball against a wall and lean against it so that the ball fits nicely in your low back and you feel supported.

2. Start with feet about 3 feet from the wall, having them wider than shoulder width apart and turn the toes out approximately 15 degrees, knee tracking over the second toe, as in figure 29A. Lift your chest.

3. Inhale, belly button in lightly and hold (this helps create a corset effect on the spine, stiffening the spine and protecting it). If you begin cramping, simply contract your pelvic floor (pretend you are stopping yourself from urinating) and focus on using the buttocks and thighs to protect your back, figure 29A.

4. Bending from the knees, roll the ball down the wall, slowly sitting into a squat. Keep your chest lifted, eyes on the horizon and shoulder blades pulled together, figure 29B.

5. Go as far as you can while maintaining a 35 degree lumbar curve, keeping your shin vertical (do not let your knee go over your toes). Stop when you feel you are about to lose your curve and feel your back muscles working too hard.

6. As you come up out of the movement, press through your heels and slowly exhale through pursed lips.

## Modifications:

1. If you want a challenge, you can perform this exercise with one leg at a time.

2. This exercise can also be done holding your baby postpartum.

## Variables:

| | |
|---|---|
| Reps: | 8-12 |
| Sets: | 1-3 |
| Tempo: | 3-1-3 |
| Intensity: | -2 reps (stop when you can do 2 more reps with good form) |
| Rest: | 60-90 sec. |

## Benefits:

1. This exercise provides excellent lifting mechanics as well as strengthening all the structures that support the pelvis and back. In addition, it helps to stabilize the sacroiliac joint.

# STATIC LUNGE

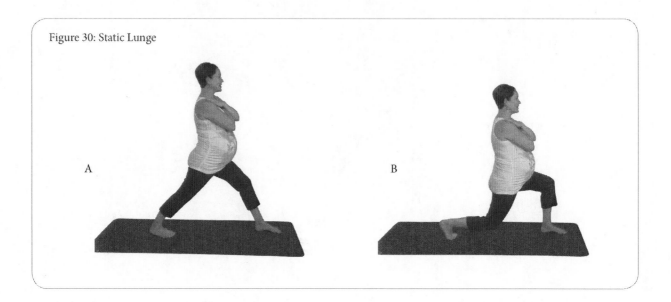

Figure 30: Static Lunge

A

B

## Cues:

1. Start with feet shoulder width apart and step one foot back about 2-3 feet, making sure that you keep your feet shoulder width apart and toes pointing forward, figure 30A.

2. Inhale, belly button in and hold (this helps create a corset effect on the spine, stiffening the spine and protecting it). If you have abdominal cramps, simply contract your pelvic floor (pretend you are stopping yourself from urinating) and focus on using the buttocks and thighs to protect your back.

3. Bending from the knees, drop your back knee toward the floor, keeping the front shin vertical as in figure 30B.

4. Go as far as you can while maintain a 35 degree lumbar curve, keeping your front shin vertical (do not let your knee go over your toes). Stop when you feel you are about to lose your curve and feel your back muscles working too hard.

5. As you come up out of the movement, press through your front heel, squeezing both buttocks and slowly exhale through pursed lips.

## Modifications:

1. If you have a hard time balancing, hold onto a stick or the edge of a chair.

2. This exercise can also be done while holding your baby postpartum.

## Variables:

Reps:  8-12 each leg

Sets:  1-3

Tempo:  3-1-3

Intensity:  -2 reps (stop when you can do 2 more reps with good form)

Rest:  60-90 sec.

## Benefits:

1. This exercise strengthens the buttocks and thighs and will teach you proper exercise technique when lunging to pick up your baby.

# HIP EXTENSION FROM THE FLOOR

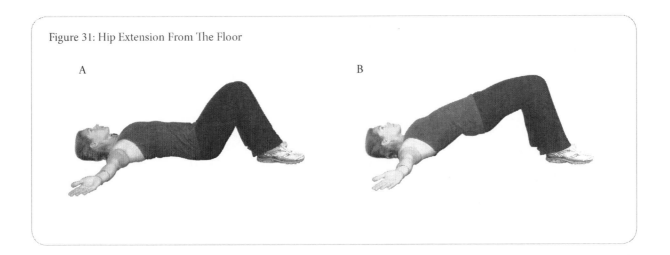

Figure 31: Hip Extension From The Floor

A                    B

## Cues:

1. Lie on your back, palms facing the ceiling, feet shoulder width apart and neck long, pressing the back of your head into the floor, figure 31A.

2. Press your hips up, starting the movement with your buttocks, keeping the chest open and neck long, figure 31B. Make sure your knee is tracking over the second toe and the shins are vertical.

## Precautions:

1. If you feel this in the low back, really squeeze your buttocks and lower the hips slightly.

2. If you feel pain in your neck, place a small rolled up towel under your neck.

3. If lying on your back causes you to feel dizzy or uncomfortable do not perform exercises on your back.

## Modifications:

1. To help open your chest, clasp your hands under your body.

2. This exercise can also be done with your baby on your belly postpartum.

## Variables:

Reps: 8-12

Sets: 1-3

Tempo: 3-1-3

Intensity: -2 reps (stop when you can do 2 more reps with good form)

Rest: 60-90 sec.

## Benefits:

1. This exercise strengthens the buttocks and thighs and will teach you proper exercise technique for the squat.

# SWISS BALL HIP EXTENSION BACK ON BALL

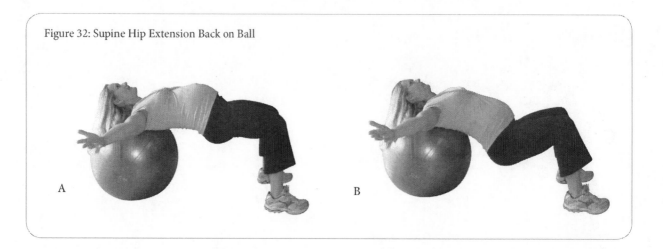

Figure 32: Supine Hip Extension Back on Ball

A

B

## Cues:

1. Lie on a Swiss ball with your head and neck fully supported, neck in neutral. Your palms are facing the ceiling, feet shoulder width apart.

2. Press your hips up starting the movement with your buttocks, keeping the chest open and neck long, figure 32A. Make sure your knee is tracking over the second toe and the shins are vertical.

3. Drop your hips toward the floor, without letting the ball move, keeping your shins vertical, figure 32B.

4. Press slowly back up to the start position, without pushing the ball forward or backward.

## Precautions:

1. If you feel this in the low back, really squeeze your buttocks and do not come up too high in the movement.

2. If you feel pain in your neck, make sure your head is not falling back over the ball, or that your chin is not buried in your chest.

## Modifications:

1. To make this exercise harder, you can do a hip extension with one leg at a time. If you choose to do this, make sure your hands are near the floor should you start to fall to one side or, hold a dumbbell vertical in each hand so they are on the floor, giving you stability.

2. This exercise can also be done with your baby on your belly postpartum.

## Variables:

Reps: 8-12

Sets: 1-3

Tempo: 3-1-3

Intensity: -2 reps (stop when you can do 2 more reps with good form)

Rest: 60-90 sec.

## Benefits:

1. Strengthens the glutes, hamstrings and quadriceps, as well as activating the nervous system to help with balance and stability.

# TOE TOUCH DRILL

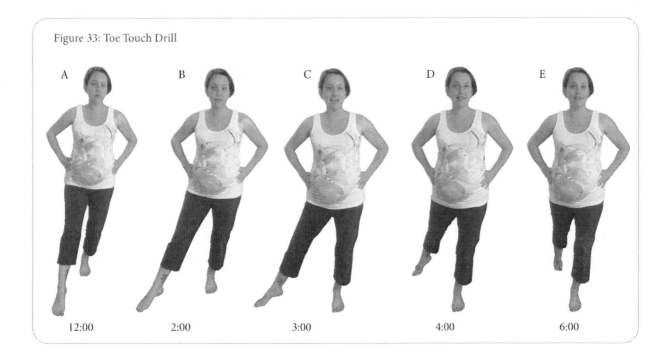

Figure 33: Toe Touch Drill

A    12:00    B    2:00    C    3:00    D    4:00    E    6:00

## Cues:

1. Stand facing a mirror with feet shoulder width apart, hands on the top of the pelvis to make sure it stays neutral and does not tip forward or backward, figure 33A.

2. Bend the left leg to about 20 degrees or as much as you can without letting the knee come past the toes. Make sure the knee is tracking over the second toe from the big toe. Hold this position.

3. With the right leg, slowly touch out to the front as if touching your toe around a clock, starting with 12:00, figure 33A, bring the foot back, then touch 2:00 (45 degrees), figure 33B, then touch 3:00 (out to side), figure 33C, then touch 4:00 (45 degrees back), figure 33D and then straight back to 6:00, figure 33E. The left leg stays bent, holding the starting position the entire time.

4. Continue to do this for 30 - 60 seconds then repeat on other side.

## Precautions:

1. If you feel this in your knee, do not go as deep into the knee bend.

2. If you feel pain in your back, squeeze your glutes and make sure your tail bone is tucked under.

## Modifications:

1. This exercise can be done by touching in front of you and as you come back to start, releasing the bend in the knee for a second or two and then bend the knee again and touch the next place on the clock.

## Variables:

Reps:  1 with a 30-60 second hold tempo or 5-15 reps per leg when not holding.

Tempo:  30-60 seconds per leg or 5-15 reps per leg with a 2-1-2 tempo

Rest:  60-90 seconds

Sets:  1-3

Intensity:  -5 seconds (stop when you feel you can hold it 5 more seconds) or -1 rep

## Benefits:

1. Strengthens the glutes and quadriceps, as well as teaching the knee how to track properly. This is an excellent exercise for those who have trouble keeping the knee tracking over the second toe during a lunge, squat or when walking or running.

# SUPINE HIP EXTENSION FEET ON BALL

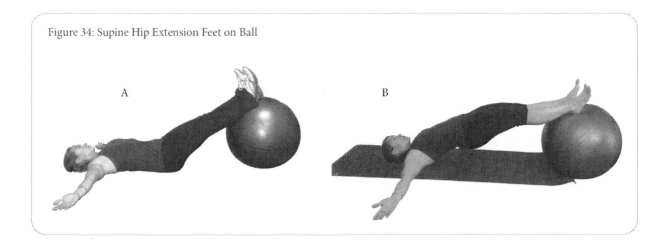

Figure 34: Supine Hip Extension Feet on Ball

A

B

## Cues:

1. Lie on the floor with your palms facing the ceiling and place your heels on a Swiss ball, figure 34A.

2. Slowly press the hips up using your rear end to start the movement and stopping when your hips are flat like a table top, figure 34B.

3. Slowly lower back to the ground.

## Variables:

Reps: 6-12

Sets: 1-3

Tempo: 2-2-2

Intensity: -2 reps (stop when you can do 2 more reps with good form)

Rest: 60-90 sec.

## Precautions:

1. If you feel pain in your back, squeeze your glutes and make sure your hips are not pushing up too high into the movement, over arching your back.

## Benefits:

1. Strengthens the glutes and hamstrings as well as the nervous system.

## Modifications:

1. You can do this same exercise with a chair.

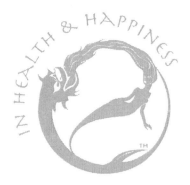

IN HEALTH & HAPPINESS

# BACK

# BENT-OVER-ROW

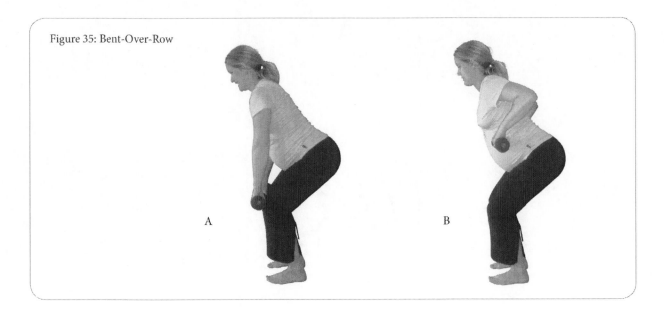

Figure 35: Bent-Over-Row

A

B

## Cues:

1. Stand with feet shoulder width apart and head in neutral while looking at the floor about 2-3 feet in front of you. Hold a dumbbell in each hand, at knee level. Knees are bent to about 20 degrees and belly button is drawn in lightly as in figure 35A.

2. Start the movement by squeezing your shoulder blades together as you pull the weight up toward the bottom of your rib cage as in figure 35B. Hold for 2 seconds and slowly lower. For this exercise you will inhale as you pull and exhale as you release, because inhalation is coupled with extension.

## Precautions:

1. If you feel pain in your back, this exercise can be done in a lunge stance or with one arm at a time, while placing the other hand on a bench for support.

## Modifications:

1. This can also be done standing on a Bosu ball for an added challenge.

## Variables:

| | |
|---|---|
| Reps: | 8-12 |
| Sets: | 1-3 |
| Tempo: | 2-2-2 |
| Intensity: | -2 reps (stop when you can do 2 more reps with good form) |
| Rest: | 60-90 sec. |

## Benefits:

1. Strengthens the upper back to help improve posture and holds the chest up as the breasts get heavier.

2. This is an important exercise to get you ready for holding a baby for long periods of time.

# SEATED ROW WITH TUBING

## Cues:

1. Sit on the floor with your chest lifted and knees bent to about 20 degrees, belly button is drawn in lightly.

2. Wrap the tube around the bottom of the feet in order to create tension in the tube. You do not want the tube to be loose.

3. Start the movement by squeezing your shoulder blades together as you pull the tube toward the bottom of your rib cage, figure 36. Hold for 2 seconds and slowly release. For this exercise you will inhale as you pull and exhale as you release, because inhalation is coupled with extension.

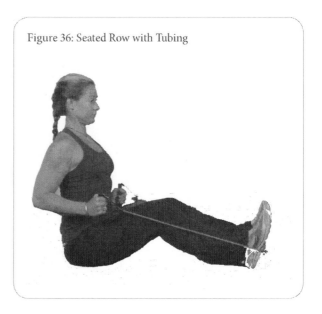

Figure 36: Seated Row with Tubing

## Variables:

|  |  |
|---|---|
| Reps: | 8-12 |
| Sets: | 1-3 |
| Tempo: | 2-2-2 |
| Intensity: | -2 reps (stop when you can do 2 more reps with good form) |
| Rest: | 60-90 sec. |

## Benefits:

1. Strengthens the upper back to help improve posture and holds the chest up as the breasts get heavier.

2. This is an important exercise to get you ready for holding a baby for long periods of time.

# SUPERWOMAN

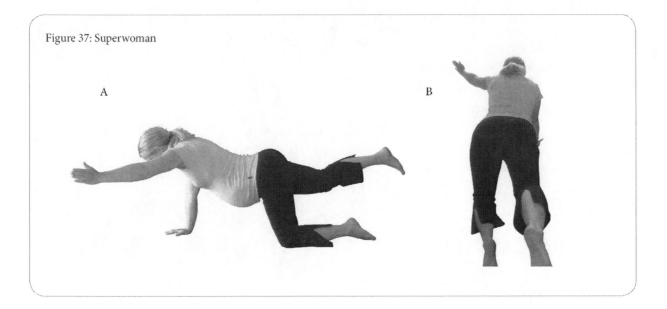

Figure 37: Superwoman

A

B

## Cues:

1. From a table top position, slowly raise one leg to about parallel to the floor as you raise the opposite arm up at a 45 degree angle, thumb to the ceiling, figure 37 A&B.

2. Keep your belly button drawn in lightly.

3. Hold for 2 seconds, lower and change sides.

## Modifications:

1. If it is difficult to keep your balance, simply alternate lifting just the legs until you find your balance, then add the arm.

## Benefits:

1. Strengthens and coordinates the upper and lower body as well as the right and left side of the body in a functional movement pattern similar to gait (walking).

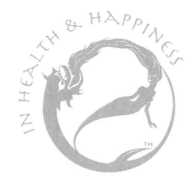

IN HEALTH & HAPPINESS

CHEST

# WALL PUSH-UP

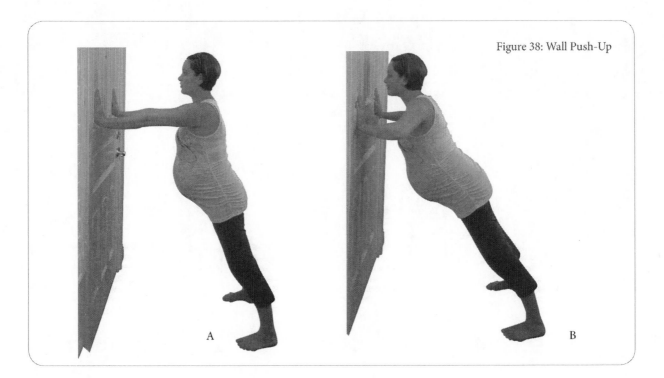

Figure 38: Wall Push-Up

## Cues:

1. Stand with your palms flat on the wall at shoulder height as in figure 38A.

2. Looking straight ahead, neck in neutral, drawing your belly button lightly and slowly lower your chest toward the wall or door keeping the head in line with your hips at all times, figure 38B.

3. Press back up to the start position finishing the push up so that your shoulder blades are flat on your back.

## Modifications:

1. If this bothers your back, you can do the push up from your hip as on page 75.

## Variables:

Reps: 8-12

Sets: 1-3

Tempo: 2-2-2

Intensity: -2 reps (stop when you can do 2 more reps with good form)

Rest: 60-90 sec.

## Benefits:

1. Strengthens the chest and arms.

# PUSH UP

## Cues:

1. Kneel on the floor making sure the top of your thigh, not your knee cap, is on the floor, figure 39A.

2. Your hands should be about shoulder width apart and directly under your shoulders, neck in neutral. Draw your belly button in lightly and slowly lower your chest toward the floor, keeping the head in line with your hips at all times, figure 39B.

3. Press back up to the start position, finishing the push up so that your shoulder blades are flat on your back.

## Modifications:

1. If this bothers your back you can do the push up against a wall as seen on page 74, or from the hips, as in figure 40A&B.

## Variables:

| | |
|---|---|
| Reps: | 8-12 |
| Sets: | 1-3 |
| Tempo: | 2-2-2 |
| Intensity: | -2 reps (stop when you can do 2 more reps with good form) |
| Rest: | 60-90 sec. |

## Benefits:

1. Strengthens the chest and arms.

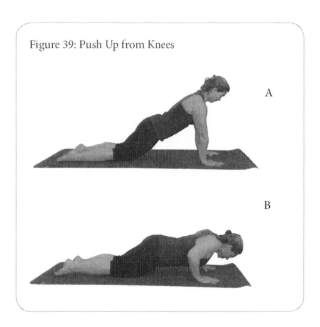

Figure 39: Push Up from Knees

A

B

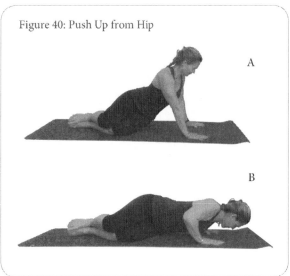

Figure 40: Push Up from Hip

A

B

# BOSU BALL PUSH-UP

Figure 41: Bosu Ball Push-Up

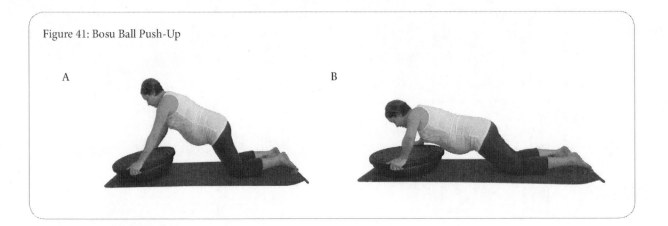

A                B

## Cues:

1. Kneel on the floor making sure the top of your thighs, not your knee caps, are on the floor, figure 41A.

2. Grab the outside of the Bosu ball where there are small handles, neck in neutral. Draw your belly button in lightly and slowly lower your chest toward the Bosu ball, keeping the head in line with your hips at all times, figure 41B.

3. Press back up to the start position, finishing the push up so that your shoulder blades are flat on your back.

## Modifications:

1. This exercise can also be done from the floor if it is too intense using the Bosu ball.

## Variables:

Reps: 8-12

Sets: 1-3

Tempo: 2-2-2

Intensity: -2 reps (stop when you can do 2 more reps with good form)

Rest: 60-90 sec.

## Benefits:

1. Strengthens the chest and arms as well as developing the nervous system on an unstable surface.

# BENCH PRESS FROM FLOOR

## Cues:

1. Lie on the floor with one dumbbell in each hand, holding the dumbbell horizontal next to your chest, figure 42A.

2. Slowly press the dumbbells up until they are above the chest, not the face.

3. Lower back to the start position.

## Modifications:

1. This exercise can also be done holding the dumbbells vertical to develop wrist strength, figure 42B.

2. Once the wrists are strong enough, this exercise can be done holding kettle bells either with the flat side in your hands or holding onto the handles as in figure 42C.

## Variables:

Reps: 8-12

Sets: 1-3

Tempo: 2-2-2

Intensity: -2 reps (stop when you can do 2 more reps with good form)

Rest: 60-90 sec.

## Benefits:

1. Strengthens the chest, arms and wrists, while protecting the shoulders by not allowing the arms to drop back too far into the down position. Once the baby arrives, your wrists will become very sore holding the baby, so it is important to continue to build wrist strength.

## Precautions:

1. If lying on your back causes you to feel dizzy or uncomfortable do not perform exercises on your back.

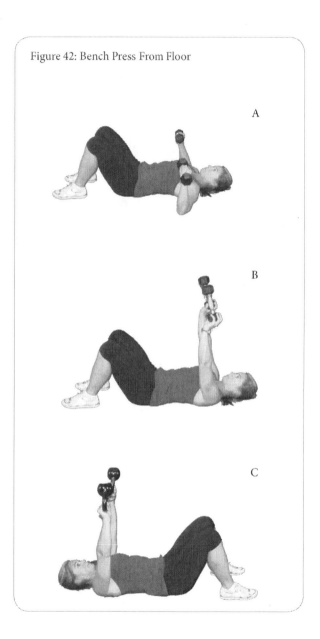

Figure 42: Bench Press From Floor

A

B

C

# SWISS BALL CHEST PRESS

## Cues:

1. Lie on a Swiss ball, making sure the head and neck are fully supported, with one dumbbell in each hand, holding the dumbbell horizontal next to your chest, figure 43A.

2. Slowly press the dumbbells up until they are above the chest, not the face, figure 43B.

3. Lower back to the start position.

## Modifications:

1. This exercise can also be done holding the dumbbells vertical to develop wrist strength, figure 43C.

2. Once the wrists are strong enough, this exercise can be done holding kettle bells, either with the flat side in your hands, or holding onto the handles as shown on page 87.

## Variables:

|   |   |
|---|---|
| Reps: | 8-12 |
| Sets: | 1-3 |
| Tempo: | 2-2-2 |
| Intensity: | -2 reps (stop when you can do 2 more reps with good form) |
| Rest: | 60-90 sec. |

## Benefits:

1. Strengthens the chest, arms and wrists, while protecting the shoulders, by not allowing the arms to drop back too far into the down position. By using the Swiss ball, you are integrating the entire body into the movement pattern, strengthening the legs and core at the same time.

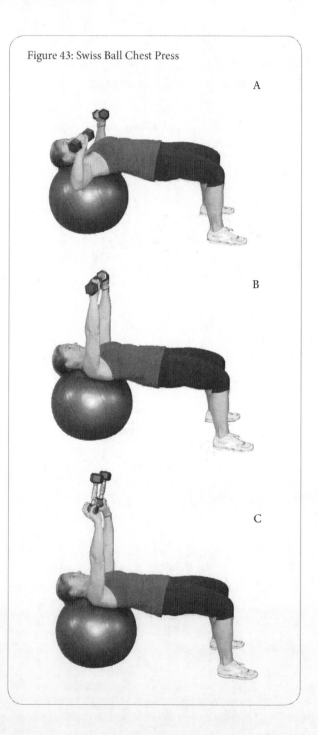

Figure 43: Swiss Ball Chest Press

A

B

C

# SWISS BALL CHEST FLY

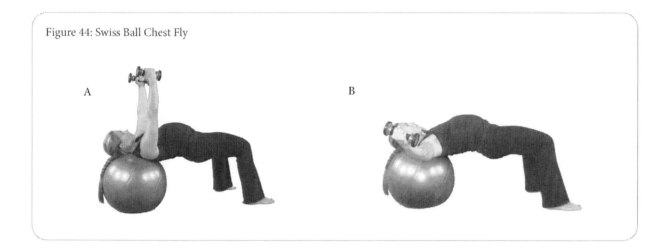

Figure 44: Swiss Ball Chest Fly

A

B

## Cues:

1. Lie on a Swiss ball, making sure the head and neck are fully supported, with one dumbbell in each hand, holding the dumbbells horizontal, with arms held up straight, right above the chest, figure 44A.

2. Slowly lower the dumbbells out to the side as you bend the elbows slightly, figure 44B.

3. Using the chest muscles, squeeze the chest and bring the dumbbells back to the start position.

## Modifications:

1. This exercise can also be done on the floor to decrease the intensity.

## Variables:

Reps:       8-12

Sets:       1-3

Tempo:      2-2-2

Intensity:  -2 reps (stop when you can do 2 more reps with good form)

Rest:       60-90 sec.

## Benefits:

1. Strengthens the chest, arms and wrists, while protecting the shoulders, by not allowing the arms to drop back too far into the down position. By using the Swiss ball you are integrating the entire body into the movement pattern, strengthening the legs, back and core at the same time.

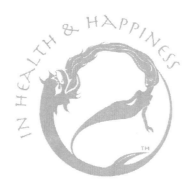

IN HEALTH & HAPPINESS

# ARMS & BALANCING

# STANDING BOSU BALL BICEPS CURL

## Cues:

1. Stand on a Bosu ball or the floor with feet about shoulder width apart, holding a dumbbell in each hand.

2. Slowly curl the dumbbells, making sure to keep your wrists straight, figure 45.

3. Lower back to the start position.

## Modifications:

1. This exercise can also be done standing on the floor or seated to reduce the intensity.

## Variables:

| | |
|---|---|
| Reps: | 8-12 |
| Sets: | 1-3 |
| Tempo: | 2-2-2 |
| Intensity: | -2 reps (stop when you can do 2 more reps with good form) |
| Rest: | 60-90 sec. |

## Benefits:

1. Strengthens the arms and by using the Bosu ball you are integrating the entire body into the movement pattern, strengthening the legs, back and core at the same time. This is ideal for keeping your strength up so that you can pick your baby up easily.

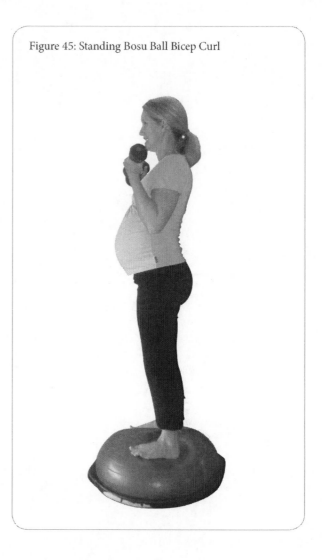

Figure 45: Standing Bosu Ball Bicep Curl

# STANDING BOSU BALL TRICEP EXTENSION

## Cues:

1. Stand on a Bosu ball or the floor with feet about shoulder width apart, with a dumbbell in each hand.

2. Raise the arms with bent elbows close to the ears and slowly extend the elbows up, allowing the elbows to fall into a natural position, figure 46.

3. Lower back to the start position.

## Modifications:

1. This exercise can also be done standing on the floor or seated to reduce the intensity.

## Variables:

Reps: 8-12

Sets: 1-3

Tempo: 2-2-2

Intensity: -2 reps (stop when you can do 2 more reps with good form)

Rest: 60-90 sec.

## Benefits:

1. Strengthens the arms and by using the Bosu ball you are integrating the entire body into the movement pattern, strengthening the legs, back and core at the same time.

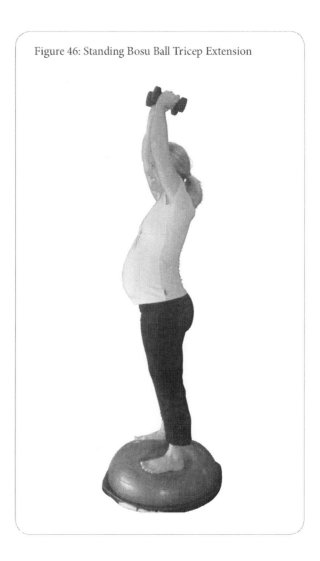

Figure 46: Standing Bosu Ball Tricep Extension

# STANDING AIREX PAD BICEP TRICEP

## Cues:

1. Stand on an Airex Pad or the floor with feet about shoulder width apart, holding a dumbbell in each hand.

2. Hold the left dumbbell down at your side and the right dumbbell up over the head, with the elbow bent as in figure 47A.

3. Slowly curl the dumbbell in the left hand as you extend the elbow on the right arm, as in figure 47B.

4. Make sure to keep your wrist straight.

5. Lower back to the start position.

6. Repeat for 12-15 reps and switch sides.

## Modifications:

1. This exercise can also be done standing on the floor or seated to reduce the intensity.

2. You can increase the intensity by standing on a Bosu ball.

## Variables:

| | |
|---|---|
| Reps: | 12-15 |
| Sets: | 1-3 |
| Tempo: | 2-2-2 |
| Intensity: | -2 reps (stop when you can do 2 more reps with good form) |
| Rest: | 60-90 sec. |

## Benefits:

1. Strengthens the arms and increases coordination and by using the Airex Pad you are integrating the entire body into the movement pattern, strengthening the legs, back and core at the same time. This is ideal for keeping your strength up so that you can pick your baby up easily.

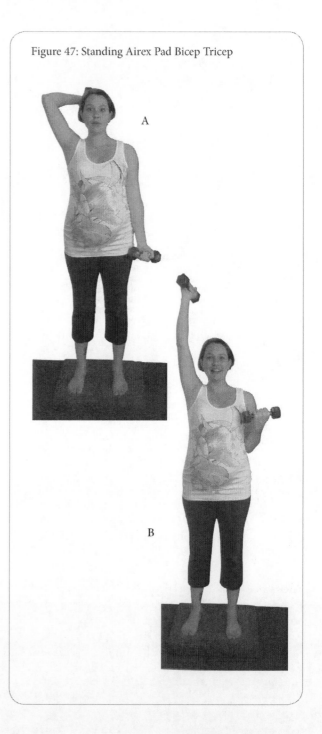

Figure 47: Standing Airex Pad Bicep Tricep

# STANDING TRICEP KICK BACK

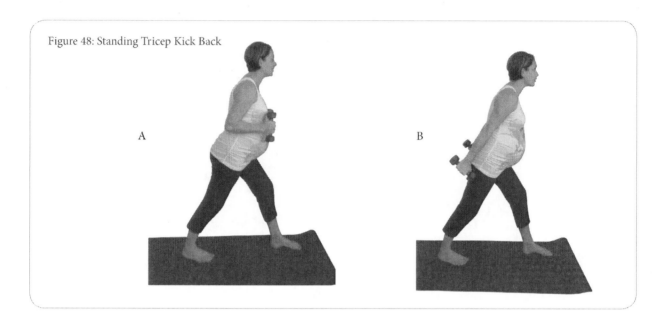

Figure 48: Standing Tricep Kick Back

A

B

## Cues:

1. Stand on the floor with feet about shoulder width apart and step one foot back about 2 feet, holding a dumbbell in each hand.

2. Lean forward slightly and bend the elbows, keeping the elbows close to your side, figure 48A.

3. Slowly extend the elbows and as you press the dumbbells back, extend the arm to a comfortable position, figure 48B.

4. Return to the start position.

## Modifications:

1. This exercise can also be done seated to reduce the intensity.

## Variables:

Reps: 8-12

Sets: 1-3

Tempo: 2-2-2

Intensity: -2 reps (stop when you can do 2 more reps with good form)

Rest: 60-90 sec.

## Benefits:

1. Strengthens the back of the arms.

# SWISS BALL WRIST PRESS

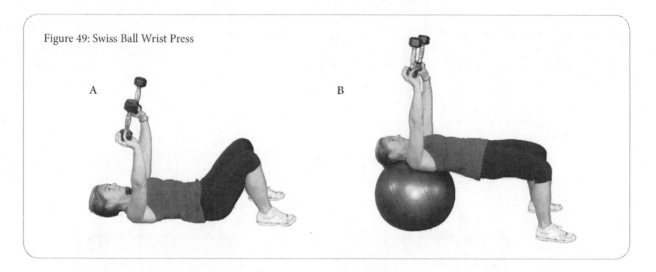

Figure 49: Swiss Ball Wrist Press

A

B

## Cues:

1. Lie on the floor with one dumbbell in each hand, holding the dumbbell vertical next to your chest.

2. Slowly press the dumbbells up until they are directly above the chest, not the face, figure 49A.

3. Lower back to the start position.

## Modifications:

1. This exercise can also be done on a Swiss ball. Make sure the head and shoulders are completely supported when lying on the Swiss ball, figure 49B.

2. Once the wrists are strong enough, this exercise can be done holding kettle bells, either with the flat side in your hands, figure 50A or holding onto the handles as in figure 50B.

3. Please note that these are wrist exercises, so choose a weight that is light and easy for the wrists to control.

## Variables:

Reps:  8-12

Sets:  1-3

Tempo:  2-2-2

Intensity:  -2 reps (stop when you can do 2 more reps with good form)

Rest:  60-90 sec.

## Benefits:

1. Strengthens the chest, arms and wrists, while protecting the shoulders by not allowing the arms to drop back too far into the down position. By using the Swiss ball you are integrating the entire body into the movement pattern, strengthening the legs, back and core at the same time.

# SWISS BALL KETTLE BELL WRIST PRESS

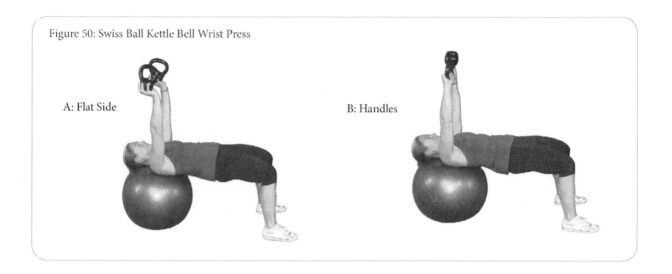

Figure 50: Swiss Ball Kettle Bell Wrist Press

A: Flat Side

B: Handles

# POWER WEB WRIST EXERCISE

## Cues:

1. Stand with feet about shoulder width apart, holding a power web in one hand.

2. Raise the arm out in front of you and squeeze the fingers together and then spread them apart 8-12 times, figure 51.

3. Repeat on other side.

## Modifications:

1. This exercise can also be done standing on a Bosu ball or seated on a Swiss ball.

## Variables:

Reps: 8-12

Sets: 1-3

Tempo: 2-2-2

Intensity: -2 reps (stop when you can do 2 more reps with good form)

Rest: 60-90 sec.

## Benefits:

1. Strengthens the wrists and hand grip.

Power webs are sold at www.fitter1.com.

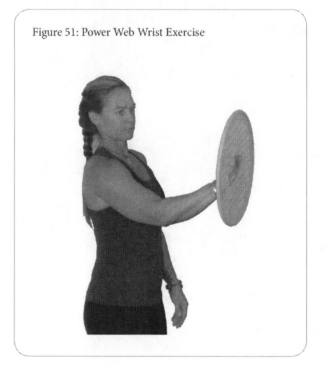

Figure 51: Power Web Wrist Exercise

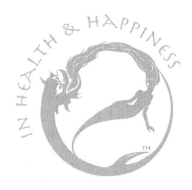

# CORE

# FORWARD BALL ROLL

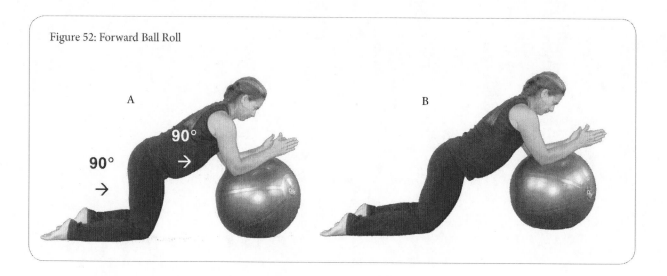

Figure 52: Forward Ball Roll

A

B

## Cues:

1. Start with knees on a mat or soft surface and fore-arms on a Swiss ball, as in figure 52A.

2. Make sure your arms are at a 90 degree angle to the torso and the hips are at a 90 degree angle. Your head should be in line with your shoulders and hips, as if you had a stick on your back, figure 52A.

3. Draw your belly button in just enough to slim your waistline slightly (do not round your back). If your abdominals cramps, contract your pelvic floor. Holding this position, slowly extend the arms and hips forward, moving at the same pace.

4. Go as far as you can while keeping good alignment and maintaining a 35 degree lumbar curve, figure 52B. Be sure to keep the tongue on the roof of the mouth.

5. Once you hit your end point (this is when you can no longer maintain a 35 degree lumbar curve) slowly roll back to the start position. It is important not to push yourself into poor form as you will create further imbalances in the body.

## Modifications:

1. Relax your belly if you feel cramping.

2. If you have difficulty holding a neutral spine place a dowel rod (6' x 1 3/8") on your back as a cue for where your body alignment should be.

## Variables:

Reps:   6-12

Sets:   1-3

Tempo:   3-3-3

Intensity:   -2 reps (stop when you can do 2 more reps with good form)

Rest:   60-90 sec.

## Benefits:

1. This is an excellent exercise to train the core and the extensor and flexor chain of the body. It helps balance the neck extensors and flexors with the torso extensors and flexors and the hip extensors and flexors, thereby creating good posture.

# TUMMY VACUUM

## Cues:

1. Start on all fours, with the knees under the hips and the hands under the shoulders, as in figure 53.

2. Make sure that your arms are at a 90 degree angle to the torso and the hips are at a 90 degree angle. You head should be in line with your shoulders and hips, as if you had a stick on your back, figure 53.

3. Draw your belly button in just enough to slim your waistline slightly (do not round your back). If your abdominals cramp, contract your pelvic floor. Hold this position for 10 seconds and then relax for 10 seconds, without letting the low back sag.

4. It is important the there is no change in your upper back as you perform this exercise.

Figure 53: Tummy Vacuum

## Modifications:

1. If you have difficulty holding a neutral spine, place a dowel rod (6' x 1 3/8") on your back, as a cue for where your body alignment should be.

## Variables:

| | |
|---|---|
| Reps: | 10 |
| Sets: | 1-3 |
| Tempo: | 10 seconds on 10 seconds off |
| Intensity: | -2 reps (stop when you can do 2 more reps with good form) |
| Rest: | 60-90 sec. |

## Benefits:

1. This is an excellent exercise to train the transversus abdominis, (core) while maintaining good posture.

# SWISS BALL PELVIC TILT

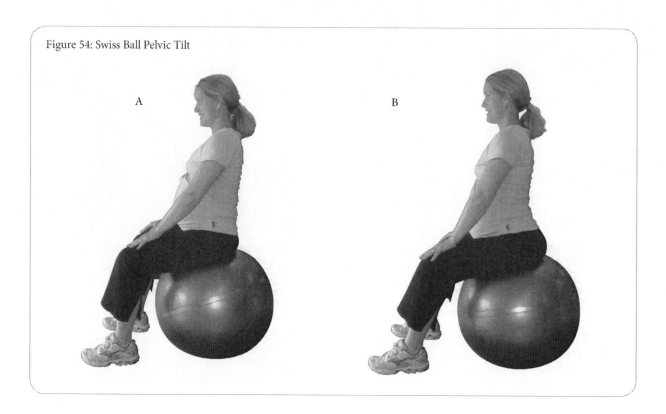

Figure 54: Swiss Ball Pelvic Tilt

A          B

## Cues:

1. Sit on a Swiss ball with your chest lifted and eyes on the horizon. Make sure your thighs are parallel to the floor or slightly higher.

2. Tuck your tail under and move the Swiss ball toward your feet, figure 54A.

3. Next, tilt your pelvis forward moving the Swiss ball away from your feet, figure 54B.

## Variables:

    Reps:  10-20

    Sets:  1-3

    Tempo:  3-3-3

    Intensity:  -2 reps (stop when you can do 2 more reps with good form)

    Rest:  60-90 sec.

## Benefits:

1. This is an excellent exercise to open the hips and take stress off the low back.

# KEGELS

## Muscles of the Pelvic Floor

*superior view*

Pubic bone

Inguinal ligament

Deep dorsal vein of clitoris
Urethra
Vaginal canal
Rectum

Levator ani muscle
Pubococcygeus
Iliococcygeus
Ischio-coccygeus

Ischial spine

Coccyx

Piriformis muscle

Sacral promontory

Illustration 7:
Muscles of the Pelvic Floor © Anatomy Coloring Book

## How to do kegel exercises

**It takes diligence to identify your pelvic floor muscles and learn how to contract and relax them. Here are some pointers:**

Find the right muscles by trying to stop the flow of urine when you urinate. If you succeed, you've got the basic move. Don't make a habit of starting and stopping your urine stream though. Doing Kegel exercises with a full bladder or while emptying your bladder can actually weaken the muscles, as well as lead to incomplete emptying of the bladder, which increases the risk of a urinary tract infection.

Once you've identified your pelvic floor muscles, empty your bladder and sit or lie down. Contract your pelvic floor muscles, hold the contraction for five seconds, then relax for five seconds. Try it four or five times in a row. Work up to keeping the muscles contracted for 10 seconds at a time, relaxing for 10 seconds between contractions. Maintain your focus. For best results, focus on tightening only your pelvic floor muscles. Be careful not to flex the muscles in your abdomen, thighs or buttocks. Avoid holding your breath. Instead, breathe freely during the exercises. Repeat three times a day. Aim for at least three sets of 10 repetitions a day. You might make a practice of fitting in a set every time you do a routine task, such as checking e-mail, commuting to work, preparing meals or watching TV.

# CRUNCH TO REPAIR ABDOMINAL WALL SPLIT (DIASTASIS RECTI)

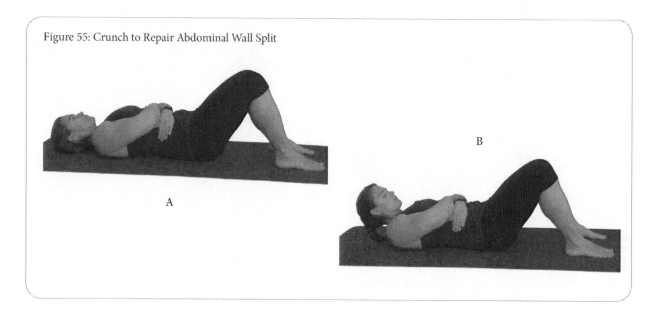

Figure 55: Crunch to Repair Abdominal Wall Split

## Cues:

1. Lie on the floor and hold the abdominal wall where it has split with your hands crossed over your abdomen and pull tightly, figure 55A.

2. Place the tongue on the roof of your mouth just behind the top teeth.

3. First, just lift your head and neck off the floor slowly as you exhale, figure 55B. If nothing is forcing it's way out of the gap, then raise your shoulders off the floor, making sure the gap stays closed and nothing is bulging out.

4. Perform this a few times a day if you are pregnant to discourage further separation and 50 times a day in sets of 10 each few hours postpartum. Continue to do this for about one week and the gap should begin to close.

5. Be mindful to perform this exercise slowly.

## Modifications:

1. Remember, if you do not have diastasis recti, crunches should not be performed as your belly becomes larger or you may create a splitting of the abdominal wall.

## Variables:

Reps: A few times a day prenatal and up to 50 a day postpartum.

Sets: 1-3

Tempo: 3-3-3

Intensity: -2 reps (stop when you can do 2 more reps with good form)

Rest: 60-90 sec.

## Benefits:
1. This exercise will help close a wide gap in the abdominal wall.

## Precautions:

1. If lying on your back causes you to feel dizzy or uncomfortable do not perform exercises on your back.

# LOWER ABDOMINAL #1

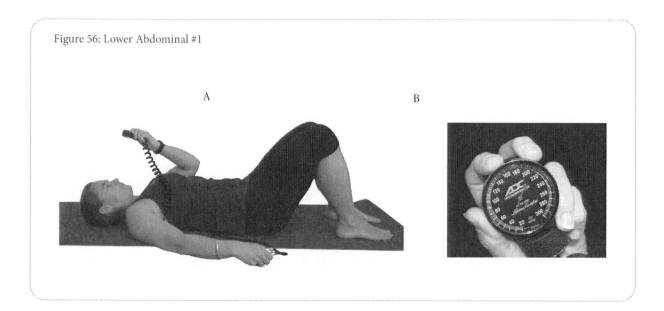

Figure 56: Lower Abdominal #1

A

B

## Cues:

1. Lie on your back with a neck roll if needed and place your hand under your back to find neutral spine (hand should fit comfortable under the back).

2. Place blood pressure cuff under back and pump it up until it fills the gap your hand filled, getting your back to neutral spine (35 degree curve), figure 56A.

3. Now put in 30 mmHg of pressure, make note what that number is, figure 56B.

4. Draw your belly button to the spine and try to increase the pressure by 30 mmHg and hold for 10 seconds.

5. Relax for 10 seconds and repeat 10 times.

## Precautions:

1. If lying on your back causes you to feel dizzy or uncomfortable do not perform exercises on your back.

## Variables:

Reps: 10-20 total

Sets: 1-3

Tempo: 10 seconds on 10 seconds off

Intensity: -2 reps (stop when you can do 2 more reps with good form)

Rest: 60-90 sec.

## Modifications:

1. Once you can no longer lie on your back, you can do this exercise standing as in figure 57A.

## Benefits:

1. This is an excellent exercise to train the "inner unit" and lower abdominal wall, without using the hip flexors. Most lower abdominal exercises work the hip flexors more than the lower abdominals, creating anterior pelvic tilt, pronation of the lower leg and low-back pain. This will also help with incontinence.

# LOWER ABDOMINAL #2 AND 2B STANDING

Figure 57: Lower Abdominal #2 and 2B Standing

A 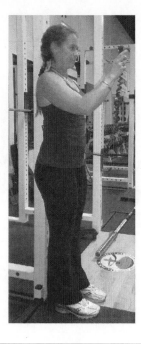 B 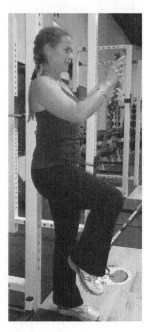 C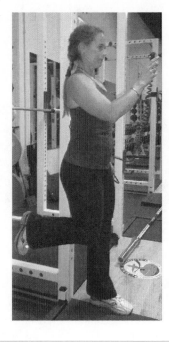

## Cues:

1. Stand against a wall or squat rack so one leg has room to move back and place your hand under your back to find neutral spine (hand should fit comfortable under the back).

2. Place blood pressure cuff under back and pump it up until it fills the gap your hand filled, getting your back to neutral spine (35 degree curve), figure 57A.

3. Now put in 30 mmHg of pressure, make note what that number is, figure 56B (the dial).

4. Draw your belly button to the spine and try to increase the pressure by 30 mmHg and hold while lifting one leg up and then the other as in figure 57B.

## Modifications:

1. To progress the exercise lift the leg and then take it behind you as in figure 57C. Perform 10-20 reps and then switch sides.

## Variables:

Reps: 10-20 total

Sets: 1-3

Tempo: 2-2-2

Intensity: -2 reps (stop when you can do 2 more reps with good form)

Rest: 60-90 sec.

## Benefits:

1. This is an excellent exercise to train the "inner unit" and lower abdominal wall, without using the hip flexors. Most lower abdominal exercises work the hip flexors more than the lower abdominals, creating anterior pelvic tilt, pronation of the lower leg and low-back pain. This will also help with incontinence.

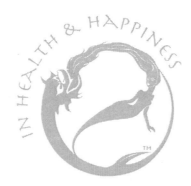

IN HEALTH & HAPPINESS

# STRENGTH TRAINING WORKOUTS

## EXERCISE PROGRAM POSTURAL

This program can be done every other day to maintain good posture throughout your pregnancy.

| Exercise | Description | Rest | Tempo | Intensity | Sets |
|---|---|---|---|---|---|
| Wall Lean page 33 | Stand with feet shoulder width apart and lean against a wall with the head, shoulders, buttocks and heels touching. Move just the buttocks and heals away from the wall 6 inches. Hold. | 60-90 sec.<br><br>**Reps**<br><br>1-3 | Up to 3 minutes | Hold as long as you can and rest 1/2 the time | 1-3 |
| Horse Stance page 34 | Get on all fours, wrists under your shoulders and knees under hips. Place a dowel rod on your back so you have 3 points of contact and lift left hand and right knee just enough to fit a piece of paper, for 10 seconds, switch sides. | **Rest**<br><br>60-90 sec.<br><br>**Reps**<br><br>10-20 Total | 10/10 | -2 reps | 1-3 |
| Kegels page 93 | Squeeze your vaginal muscles as if stopping the flow of urine. Once you identify the pelvic floor muscles, squeeze and hold for 10 seconds, then relax for 10 seconds. | **Rest**<br><br>60-90 sec.<br><br>**Reps**<br><br>5-10 | Up to 10 seconds on, rest 10 seconds | -2 reps | 1-3 |

## EXERCISE PROGRAM EASY

This program is a good overall program and should be done 1 to 3 times a week, **with a day rest in between workouts** or a light cardio workout inbetween strength training days. For detailed instruction on each exercise, refer to page number.

| Exercise | Description | Rest | Tempo | Inten-sity | Sets |
|---|---|---|---|---|---|
| Swiss Ball Wall Squat page 61 | Stand with feet wider than shoulder width, toes slightly turned out. Lean back into a Swiss ball, so it fits in the curve of your low back and squat. Make sure the knee tracks over the second toe. | 60-90 sec. / **Reps** / 8-12 | 2-2-2 | -2 reps | 1-3 |
| Hip Extension page 63 | Lie on your back and place your feet about shoulder width apart. Palms facing up arms to the side. Clasp hands under you as you press the hips up squeezing your buttocks tight. | **Rest** / 60-90 sec. / **Reps** / 8-12 | 2-2-2 | -2 reps | 1-3 |
| Seated Row with Tubing page 71 | Sit tall with knees bent and place a rubber exercise tube around feet so the tube is short. Squeeze the shoulder blades together pulling the tube toward you, hands coming to bottom of rib cage. | **Rest** / 60-90 sec. / **Reps** / 10-20 total | 2-2-2 | -2 reps | 1-3 |
| Wall Push-Up page 74 | Stand with your hands on a wall right in line with your shoulders. Slowly lower your chest toward the wall. | **Rest** / 60-90 sec. / **Reps** / 10-20 total | 2-2-2 | -2 reps | 1-3 |
| Superwoman page 72 | From all fours, raise your left arm at a 45 degree angle and lift your right leg up using your glutes. Switch sides. | **Rest** / 60-90 sec. / **Reps** / 10-20 total | 2-2-2 | -2 reps | 1-3 |

## EXERCISE PROGRAM EASY CONTINUED

This program is a good overall program and should be done 1 to 3 times a week with a day rest in between workouts or a light cardio workout in between strength training days. For detailed instruction on each exercise, refer to page number.

| Exercise | Description | Rest | Tempo | Intensity | Sets |
|---|---|---|---|---|---|
| Lower Abdominal #1 page 95 | Lie on back with knees bent and cuff under the low back opposite the belly button. Inflate until you feel pressure and add 30 mmHg. Draw your belly button in and increase the pressure by 30 mmHg. Hold for 10 seconds, relax for 10 seconds, 10-20 times. Switch to standing after the first trimester. | 60-90 sec.<br><br>**Reps**<br><br>10-20 total | 10/10 | + 30 mmHg | 1-3 |

# EXERCISE PROGRAM MODERATE

This program can be started once the easy program has been mastered for at least 3 weeks. This is a good overall program and should be done 1 to 3 times a week with a day rest in between workouts or a light cardio workout inbetwwen strength training days. For detailed instruction on each exercise refer to page number.

| Exercise | Description | Rest | Tempo | Intensity | Sets |
|---|---|---|---|---|---|
| Sumo Squat page 60 | Stand with feet wider than shoulder width, toes slightly turned out. Sit back into a squat making sure the knee tracks over the second toe. Push through the heels to return to standing. | 60-90 sec. **Reps** 8-12 | 2-2-2 | -2 reps | 1-3 |
| Swiss ball Hip Extension Back on Ball page 64 | Lie on Swiss ball, head and shoulders supported, feet about shoulder width apart. Palms facing up and arms to the side. Press the hips up, squeezing your buttocks tight. | **Rest** 60-90 sec. **Reps** 8-12 | 2-2-2 | -2 reps | 1-3 |
| Bent-Over-Row page 70 | Stand with feet shoulder width apart, knees bent to at least 20 degrees. Sit back as if squatting, making sure the knee tracks over the second toe, hands holding dumbbells at knees. Squeeze the shoulder blades together to get the back to lift the weight, bringing hands to the base of rib cage. | **Rest** 60-90 sec. **Reps** 8-12 | 2-2-2 | -2 reps | 1-3 |
| Push Up From Hip page 75 | Place your hips on the mat with hands under shoulders. Letting the elbows come out, lower into a push up position and press back up. | **Rest** 60-90 sec. **Reps** 8-12 | 2-2-2 | -2 reps | 1-3 |

# EXERCISE PROGRAM MODERATE CONTINUED

This program is a good overall program and should be done 1 to 3 times a week with a day rest in between workouts or a light cardio workout inbetween strength training days. For detailed instruction on each exercise, refer to page number.

| Exercise | Description | Rest | Tempo | Intensity | Sets |
|---|---|---|---|---|---|
| Vertical Dumbbell Press From Floor page 86 | Lie on floor, knees bent holding dumbbells vertical in your palms. Press up, keeping dumbbells directly over chest. | 60-90 sec.<br>**Reps**<br>8-12 | 2-2-2 | -2 reps | 1-3 |
| Standing Airex Pad Bicep Tricep page 84 | Stand on an airex pad, unstable surface or one leg with a dumbbell in each hand. Curl the dumbbell with one hand and try to do an overhead tricep extension with the other. | **Rest**<br>60-90 sec.<br>**Reps**<br>8-12 Each side | 2-2-2 | -2 reps | 1-3 |
| Forward Ball Roll page 90 | From all fours, place elbows on a Swiss ball with knees under hips and elbows under shoulders maintain a neutral spine. Slowly roll the ball forward until you feel you will lose form and your back wants to sag. Slowly roll back to start position. | **Rest**<br>60-90 sec.<br>**Reps**<br>8-12 | 2-2-2 | -2 reps | 1-3 |

# EXERCISE PROGRAM HARD

This program can be started once the moderate program has been mastered for at least 3 weeks. This is also is a good overall program and should be done 1 to 3 times a week with a day rest in between workouts or a light cardio workout in betwwen strength training days. For detailed instruction on each exercise refer to page number.

| Exercise | Description | Rest | Tempo | Intensity | Sets |
|---|---|---|---|---|---|
| Static Lunge page 62 | Stand with feet shoulder width apart and step one foot back about 3 feet. Bend the front knee, making sure the knee tracks over the second toe, shin stays vertical and move toward the floor dropping the back knee down. | 60-90 sec. **Reps** 8-12 Each side | 2-2-2 | -2 reps | 1-3 |
| Supine Hip Extension Feet on Ball page 67 | Lie on the floor with heels on a Swiss ball, arms out to the side palms up. Press the hips up squeezing your buttocks. Slowly release back to floor. | **Rest** 60-90 sec. **Reps** 8-12 | 2-2-2 | -2 reps | 1-3 |
| Bent-Over-Row page 70 | Stand on an unstable surface with feet shoulder width apart, knees bent to at least 20 degrees. Sit back as if squatting, making sure the knee tracks over the second toe, hands holding dumbbells at knees. Squeeze the shoulder blades together to get the back to lift the weight, bringing hands to rib cage. | **Rest** 60-90 sec. **Reps** 8-12 | 2-2-2 | -2 reps | 1-3 |
| Push Up From Knees page 75 | Place your thighs on the mat above the knee joint with hands under shoulders. Let the elbows come out as you lower into a push up position and press back up. | **Rest** 60-90 sec. **Reps** 8-12 | 2-2-2 | -2 reps | 1-3 |

# EXERCISE PROGRAM HARD CONTINUED

This program is a good overall program and should be done 1 to 3 times a week with a day rest in between workouts or a light cardio workout in between strength training days. For detailed instruction on each exercise refer to page number.

| Exercise | Description | Rest | Tempo | Intensity | Sets |
|---|---|---|---|---|---|
| Swiss Ball Wrist Press page 86 | Lie on a Swiss ball, head and shoulders supported, hips up in a table top position, holding dumbbells vertical in your palms. Press up, keeping dumbbells over chest. | 60-90 sec. **Reps** 8-12 | 2-2-2 | -2 reps | 1-3 |
| Bosu Bicep Curl page 82 | Stand on a Bosu ball, unstable surface or one leg with a dumbbell in each hand. Curl the dumbbells up. | **Rest** 60-90 sec. **Reps** 8-12 Each side | 2-2-2 | -2 reps | 1-3 |
| Tricep Kick Back page 85 | Stand in a high lunge position, holding a dumbbell in each hand, elbows bent. Lean forward slightly and press the dumbbells back with your triceps. | **Rest** 60-90 sec. **Reps** 8-12 | 2-2-2 | -2 reps | 1-3 |
| Lower Abdominal #2 Standing page 96 | Stand against a wall with a blood pressure cuff behind your low back, opposite the belly button. Pump cuff until you feel pressure and add 30 mmHg of pressure. Draw belly button in to add 30 mmHg and keep it there. Lift the right leg up with knee bent as far as you can and switch sides. | **Rest** 60-90 sec. **Reps** 10-20 total | 2-2-2 | + 30 mmHg | 1-3 |

# EXERCISE PROGRAM LOWER BODY

This program can be alternated with the upper body program to get more workouts in during the week. This program can be done at least 2 times a week but should not be done on consecutive days. Remember not to over do it. If you have a great deal of muscle soreness that does not go away, back off and move to an easier workout.

| Exercise | Description | Rest | Tempo | Intensity | Sets |
|---|---|---|---|---|---|
| Static Lunge page 62 | Stand with feet shoulder width apart and step one foot back about 3 feet. Bend the front knee, making sure the knee tracks over the second toe, the shin stays vertical and move toward the floor, dropping the back knee down. | 60-90 sec. **Reps** 8-12 Each side | 2-2-2 | -2 reps | 1-3 |
| Sumo Squat page 60 | Stand with feet wider than shoulder width apart, toes slightly turned out. Sit back into a squat making sure the knee tracks over the second toe. | **Rest** 60-90 sec. **Reps** 8-12 | 2-2-2 | -2 reps | 1-3 |
| Swiss ball Hip Extension Feet on Ball page 67 | Lie on the floor with heels on a Swiss ball, arms out to the side with palms up. Press the hips up squeezing your buttocks. Slowly lower back to the floor. | **Rest** 60-90 sec. **Reps** 8-12 | 2-2-2 | -2 reps | 1-3 |
| Lower Abdominal #2 Standing page 96 | Stand against a wall with a blood pressure cuff behind your low back opposite the belly button. Pump cuff until you feel pressure and add 30 mmHg of pressure. Lift the right leg up with knee bent as far as you can and switch sides. | **Rest** 60-90 sec. **Reps** 10-20 total | 2-2-2 | + 30 mmHG | 1-3 |

# EXERCISE PROGRAM UPPER BODY

This program can be alternated with the lower body program to get more workouts in during the week. This program can be done at least 2 times a week but should not be done on consecutive days. Remember not to over do it. If you have a great deal of muscle soreness that does not go away, back off and move to an easier workout.

| Exercise | Description | Rest | Tempo | Intensity | Sets |
|---|---|---|---|---|---|
| Bent-Over-Row page 70 | Stand with feet shoulder width apart, knees bent to at least 20 degrees. Sit back as if squatting, making sure the knee tracks over the second toe, hands holding dumbbells at knees. Squeeze the shoulder blades together to get the back to lift the weight, bringing hands to rib cage. | 60-90 sec. **Reps** 8-12 | 2-2-2 | -2 reps | 1-3 |
| Swiss Ball Wrist Press page 86 | Lie on a Swiss ball, head and shoulders supported, hips up in a table top position, holding dumbbells vertical in your palms. Press up, keeping dumbbells over chest. | **Rest** 60-90 sec. **Reps** 8-12 | 2-2-2 | -2 reps | 1-3 |
| Standing Airex Pad Bicep Tricep page 84 | Stand on an airex pad or unstable surface or one leg with a dumbbell in each hand. Curl the dumbbell with one hand and try to do an overhead tricep extension with the other. | **Rest** 60-90 sec. **Reps** 8-12 Each side | 2-2-2 | -2 reps | 1-3 |
| Forward Ball Roll page 90 | From all fours, place elbows on a Swiss ball with knees under hips and elbows under shoulders maintaining a neutral spine. Slowly roll the ball forward until just before you lose form and your back wants to sag. Slowly roll back to start position. | **Rest** 60-90 sec. **Reps** 8-12 | 2-2-2 | -2 reps | 1-3 |

# Pregnancy and Cardiovascular Exercise

## How often should you exercise and at what intensity?

You will read studies that say you can exercise at the same intensity and duration that you did prior to getting pregnant. Some studies will say to reduce your intensity to no more than a heart rate of 140 beats per minute. You will see studies that say no more than 15 minutes a day of light exercise for previously sedentary women. Regardless of what research you read, walking and aquatic exercise are two excellent tools for staying healthy and getting ready for birth.

Talk to your doctor or midwife and be smart about your exercise goals. Aerobic exercise during pregnancy is not done to lose weight. Exercise during pregnancy is to maintain your health, the baby's health and prepare your body for birth. For me, that was walking 30-60 minutes a day. My body let me know when it was too much and I took it easy. I never let my heart rate get past 140 beats per minute because I did not want to risk another miscarriage. Once again, I had to surrender. It was no longer just about me and it never will be again.

## Taking aerobic classes during pregnancy

The same rules apply with aerobic classes. Take it easy. If you love aerobic classes, try to attend at least one or two pre-natal aerobic classes a month so you can understand your limitations and hear about excellent ways to modify the exercises. These modifications should include low impact moves, minimal lateral movement if any and reduced abdominal strengthening exercises. Make sure your instructor is group fitness certified by nationally recognized organization such as the American Council on Exercise, American College of Sports Medicine, or The Cooper Institute. You can also look up instructors credentials at www.idea-fit.com.

## The benefits of exercising in the water

Swimming or attending aquatic exercise classes are extremely beneficial when you are pregnant. The buoyancy of the water takes 90 percent of your weight and you can lie on your back without the risk of supine hypotension. Water can give you 30-60 minutes of comfortable, fun exercise that can be shared with other pregnant women such as yourself. Always make sure you inquire about the credentials of your aquatic instructors. The Aquatic Exercise Association is an excellent resource for you, www.aeawave.com.

The ACOG (American Congress of Obstetricians and Gynecologists) guidelines are a good general resource for exercise and pregnancy. According to ACOG, the hormones produced during pregnancy cause the ligaments that support your joints to become relaxed. This makes the joints more mobile and more at risk for injury. The extra weight in the front of your body during pregnancy shifts your center of gravity and places stress on joints and muscles, especially those in the pelvis and lower back. This can make you less stable, cause back pain, and make you more likely to lose your balance and fall, especially in later pregnancy.

It is important to remember these guidelines during cardiovascular exercise and limit your lateral (side to side movement) as well as quick change of direction.

According to the ACOG guidelines it is important to stop exercise and call your health care provider if you have any of these symptoms:

- Vaginal bleeding
- Increased shortness of breath
- Chest pain
- Headache
- Muscle weakness
- Calf pain or swelling
- Uterine contractions
- Decreased fetal movement
- Fluid leaking from the vagina

## QUIZ #3

1. Which exercise helps strengthen the wrists in a supine position?

   _____

2. Which exercise works the pelvic floor muscles?

   _____

3. Name three exercises that help train the nervous system.

   _____, _____, _____

4. Which exercise helps balance the right and left side of the body?

   _____

5. Which exercise targets the hamstrings?

   _____

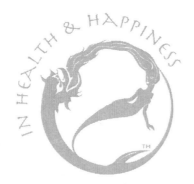

IN HEALTH & HAPPINESS

# PRENATAL YOGA

# YOGA

The yoga poses in this manual are ideal for calming the mind, opening the heart and releasing unwanted energy in the body. Yoga is an excellent way to connect to your baby and, for a short time, just surrender to the changes happening within you. Only do the poses that feel good and honor your body each and every time you practice yoga. Always remember that yoga is a balance between surrender and effort, make each pose your own.

If you practiced yoga before your pregnancy, remember that practicing yoga when you are pregnant will be very different. This is a time to nurture yourself and your baby. During pregnancy, you will need to relax your abdomen and use your back muscles during the poses that would normally require you to draw your belly button inward. Your baby needs room to grow, so allow the abdominals to become relaxed and give your baby the space it needs. For some of you, relaxing your abs is a foreign concept, one that was also very foreign to me. I had no choice, my abs began to cramp and send shooting pains throughout my body if I didn't relax my abdominal wall. This is the time to surrender and let nature take it's course. You will get those abs back and you will get that body back; all you have to do is surrender.

## YOUR YOGA PRACTICE

This section was designed to give you several prenatal yoga sequences to choose from based on your ability, needs and wants. The yoga sequences can be found starting on page 150. The pose descriptions on the sequence pages are limited, however full details of each pose are given in the yoga chapter and each pose is referenced by page number. You may simply choose to perform a pose you need for certain issue that comes up, such as low back pain or choose a sequence if you need more than just a little relief. The chart on page 111 offers pose suggestions for ailments that may be bothering you and can be addressed with just a few poses.

**When designing your own pose sequence, keep the following tips in mind:**
1. Keep the breath even on the inhale and exhales. If you lose the breath, the sequence may require too much effort and not enough surrender. For additional help with breathing see page 32.

2. Balance the body with flexion and extension. If you perform several forward folding poses in a row, balance those poses with back extension and heart opening poses.

## FINDING THE RIGHT YOGA CLASS

Yoga classes are extremely beneficial during pregnancy. Choose a class that honors pregnant women and helps you understand which poses are helpful and why; and which poses to avoid and why. Make sure that the instructor has an in-depth 200-hour yoga certification that required more than a weekend of training. In addition, it would be ideal if instructors have a group fitness certification from a nationally recognized organization such as the American Council on Exercise, The Cooper Institute or the American College of Sports Medicine.

## YOGA RESOURCES

Yoga journal (www.yogajournal.com)[23] provides some great yoga tools to help you a build your own practice. Yoga Journal was a great help in assisting me with several of the pose cues, modifications and benefits. For those who want to take yoga to the next level, "Light on Yoga" by B.K.S. Iyengar[12] is an excellent reference, known as the bible of modern yoga.

# A GUIDE TO POSES (ASANAS) THAT INCREASE STRENGTH, FLEXIBILITY AND OFFER RELIEF FROM AILMENTS AND DISEASE

One of the many benefits of yoga is that each yoga pose provides some type of relief from ailments and disease. The book "Light on Yoga" by B.K.S. Iyengar offers a wealth of information on the benefits of each asana to the mind, body and spirit. Here we will touch briefly on poses that can help with common ailments that may come up during pregnancy and postpartum. For further information, please reference the book "Light on Yoga"[12] or www.yogajournal.com[26].

## Ankles

Downward dog - page 133
Triangle - page 147
Warrior I - page 144
Warrior II - page 145
Crescent lunge - page 144
Wide-legged bend - page 141
Seated groin, hamstring , back opener - page 121

## Arms

Downward dog - page 133
Plank - page 134

## Backache

Cat and Cow - page 118
Happy baby - page 123
Hip extension - page 123
Indian squat - page 135
Legs up wall - page 124
Spinal rotation - page 128
Seated back opener - page 119
Seated forward fold - page 122
Standing or kneeling back bend - page 140
Triangle - page 147

## Balance

Tree pose - page 143

## Bladder

Cobbler's pose - page 120
Pigeon - page 130

## Constipation

All standing poses - pages 136-147
Seated forward fold  - page 122
Spinal rotations - page 128

## Digestion

Standing forward bend - page 137
Seated forward fold seated - page 122
Downward dog - page 133

## Emotions

Pigeon - page 130
Seated meditation - page 117
Triangle - page 147
Wide-legged forward bend with twist - page 142

## Flat Feet

Tree pose - page 143

## Headaches

Child's pose - page 132
Downward dog - page 133
Seated forward fold - for 5 minutes - page 122
Standing forward bend - for 3 minutes - page 137

## Hip Opener (Hips also hold emotions)

Baby cradle - page 125
Happy baby - page 123
Seated twist - page 125
Seated pretzel - page 126
Seated groin opener - page 126
Thread the needle - lower body - page 127
Figure 4 - page 128
Spinal rotation - page 128
Pigeon - page 130

## Hip, Hamstrings and Calf Stretch

Standing forward bend - page 137
Wide-legged bend - page 141
Cobbler's pose - page 120
Seated groin, hip and back opener - page 121
Leg elevation - page 124
Triangle - page 147
Happy baby - page 123
Thread the needle - lower body - page 127

## Labor Pains & Delivery

Cobbler's pose - page 120
Seated splits - page 122
Side-lying savasana - page 148

## Leg and Buttocks Strengtheners

Hip extension - page 123
Downward dog - page 133
Standing forward bend - page 137
Standing back bend - page 140
Tree pose - page 143
Wide-legged bend - page 141
Warrior I - page 144
Warrior II - page 145
Crescent lunge - page 144
Utkatasana - page 139

## Leg Cramps

Leg elevation - page 124

## Liver & Kidneys

Standing forward bend - page 137
Seated groin, hamstring and back opener - page 121
Spinal rotation - page 128
Wide-legged forward bend with twist - page 142

## Quadricep Stretch - front of thigh

Pigeon with quad stretch - page 131

## Sciatica

All standing poses - pages 136-147
Recling big toe pose - page 129
Spinal rotation - page 128
Seated forward fold - page 122
Downward dog - page 133
Baby cradle - page 125
Figure 4 - page 128

## Shoulder and Chest Stretches

Downward dog - page 133
Upward salute - page 137
Cat - page 118
Cow - page 118
Standing back bend - page 140
Wide-legged forward bend w/ hands clasped - page 142
Warrior 1 - page 144

## Shoulder, Back and Chest Strengtheners

Downward dog - page 133

## Stress Release

Seated meditation - page 117
Child's pose - page 132

## IT Band release

Figure 4 - page 128

## Wrist Strength

Downward dog - page 133
Plank - page 134

# Specific Tips For Yoga and Pregnancy

According to Iyengar[12], all the poses can be practiced the first trimester. After the first trimester, all the standing poses and the forward bends may be done with mild movements, for at this time the spine should be made strong and elastic and no pressure should be felt on the abdomen.[11] Seated forward bends may be practiced throughout the pregnancy, as these poses will strengthen the pelvic muscles and the small of the back and also reduce labor pain. Be careful not to do these poses after a meal. Other resources suggest all poses listed in this manual can be done throughout your entire pregnancy, as long as you do not feel pain. Please refer to the ACOG guidelines[2] on page 25 for when to stop exercising.

## Open your heart

During yoga, whenever possible, open your heart. Opening your heart opens your lungs and allows you to breathe. Opening your heart also allows you to open your thoughts and emotions and set your intentions for your practice.

## Using your breath

As you become aware of your breath, you will find that you can increase your energy when it is low or bring on a deep state of relaxation just by focusing on your breath. When you inhale, allow your abdomen to extend and when you exhale draw your belly button in and let out all the old air. Start to lengthen and equalize your inhale and exhale, creating a steady rhythm. Breathe in and out from the nose with the lips sealed. As you do this, start to notice a sound developing in the back of your throat like the ebb and flow of the ocean. Use counting techniques to help you focus, such as inhale up the spine for 6, hold at the top for 2 and exhale down the spine for 6. When in doubt, just breathe. Don't over think it; it takes time and practice to develop a rhythmic deep breath. See page 32 for some excellent breathing exercises.

## Neck safety

Should any pose place stress on the neck, gaze downward and place the tongue on the roof of the mouth behind your top teeth. This will activate the deep stabilizers of the neck (infra and suprahyoid muscles), giving the neck more support during your poses. I have neck issues from past car accidents and the shoulder stand places extreme pressure on my straight cervical spine. If you know you have a reverse curve or straight cervical spine avoid any poses that place pressure on the neck and head, such as shoulder stands or head stands.

## Spinal rotation and supine exercises

There has been a great deal of information out there cautioning pregnant women not to exercise lying on their back or perform side lying rotation due to the possibility of supine hypotension (a fall in blood pressure when a pregnant woman is lying on her back causing her to become dizzy and may reduce blood flow to the uterus). According to Elizabeth Noble author of Essential Exercises for the Childbearing Year, very few women experience supine hypotension during their pregnancy [18]. Consult your physician about performing back lying and spinal rotation exercises. Although many of these exercises help relieve back pain and stress placed on the hips, they may be contraindicated during your pregnancy.

## Foot placement

To protect the knee, pelvis and over all joint stability of the body, it is important to be mindful of foot placement. Page 116 offers an up close view of the foot for each foot position, based on a wall clock.

## Knee placement

The knee should always be in line with the ankle and the shin vertical in standing poses. In seated or lying poses, be sure that the knee always feels comfortable and review the modifications for any pose that places stress on your knee.

## Low back

It is important to honor your back and remember to engage the lower abdominals using a slight posterior pelvic tilt (this is a forward scooping of your tail bone under, "don't shake your tail feathers"). Remember an anterior pelvic tilt (which we do not want) is different than a forward scooping of the tail bone. When the pelvis moves anteriorly, the tail bone moves posteriorly, creating an unstable low back. You know your pelvis is moving anterior when the top of the pelvis moves toward the feet. When the top of the pelvis moves away from the feet, this is a posterior pelvic tilt. If you feel stress in your low back, tighten your glutes (buttocks) to assist your low back in supporting your body. When you are pregnant, it is very important that the glutes are toned throughout all the standing poses in order to assist the low back in supporting your body.

## Time of practice

According to Iyengar, the best time to practice yoga is in the early morning or late in the evening. "Practicing in the morning makes one work better in one's vocation. In the evening it removes the fatigue of the day's strain and makes one fresh and calm" [12].

## Use of props

It is important that you maintain proper alignment and good form during each pose in order to help your body, not hurt it.

**Blankets:**
A firm woven blanket can be folded and placed under the hips in seated positions to reduce stress on the low back and hip joints. This is ideal for women with tight hips, hamstrings and low backs.

**Straps:**
Any bath robe belt or yoga strap works well as a strap. Straps are useful to make the most out of your forward bend poses when you cannot reach your toes.

**Blocks:**
Blocks are excellent for placing under the hands in standing poses such as triangle and wide legged forward fold. Placing your hand on the blocks allows you to lengthen the back of the thighs, without placing too much stress on the muscles or joints.

**The wall:**
Most yoga poses take a great deal of balance, so use a wall to help stabilize yourself when practicing new poses for the first time. Also remember, as your baby grows, your center of gravity changes and a wall may be needed for extra support and balance.

## General positional cues:

Make each pose your own without straining or forcing the pose beyond what your body can do that day. Keep your eyes open and focus on a focal point (drishti). Be strong in your poses and contract and engage the muscles by lifting the knee caps and squeezing the shoulder blades together. During counter poses, learn to release and soften the muscles and just let go of any tightness you might have. When standing, draw the tailbone under slightly and contract the glutes to protect the back.

## Good Poses for the First Trimester

Most standing poses are fine during the first trimester. Even balance poses, such as Tree Pose, are okay provided they are done near the wall in case you lose your balance. Strengthening the leg muscles and the pelvic floor is important preparation for later phases of pregnancy; and it encourages good circulation in the legs to prevent cramping as blood pressure starts to drop. Standing twists should be avoided if they put pressure on the abdominal cavity.

Open seated twists all relieve aches in the lower back and encourage proper posture. Hip openers listed on page 111, should be a key focus because of the flexibility needed for delivery, but, be sure not to overdo it; the hormone relaxin is softening all the joints and they are easily dislocated if stretched too far. Avoid any intense abdominal work, such as Boat Pose, because of the delicate situation in the uterus.

## Contraindicated Poses

Pregnant women should avoid most inversions because you don't want to encourage circulation away from the uterus. Additionally, because of the low blood pressure pregnant women usually experience, inversions can cause dizziness. The one exception, however, is Downward Dog, which is fine for short periods of time. Because of the physical demands during the first trimester, do not do high-energy sequences, such as intense vinyasa series and Sun Salutations with jump-backs. Avoid most back bends, because they place too much stretch on the abdominal muscles. The one exception is the hip extension (Bridge Pose).

## Side-lying Savasana

A vital part of a prenatal routine is relaxation. "One thing I want every pregnant woman to do is lie down every day for 20 minutes in side-lying Savasana (Corpse Pose)," says Judith Lasater. "Rest deeply every day. Labor is the metabolic equivalent of swimming nine miles, so a mother needs to learn how to rest and listen to her body."[26]

When you are pregnant, lay on your left side for Corpse Pose at the end of class (all side-lying poses should be on the left side, to avoid pressure on the vena cava vein, which moves blood from the lower part of the body—the uterus—to the heart). Arrange blankets and bolsters under your right knee, or belly if you are starting to show), right arm, and head, so all parts of the body are supported. If you begin a habit of recuperating after physical activity now, you will fine-tune your ability to relax on cue; which is a crucial part of labor and delivery.

## Building Strength, Encouraging Rest

During the first trimester, the sensations of pregnancy are still new, so you might be tempted to overdo a sequence. Practice with a new awareness of the baby inside you and of your body's need for rest. It is now time to embrace a gentler, more introspective yoga practice.

## FOOT POSITIONS

During many of the standing poses, your feet will be in different positions to ensure your knee is aligned properly and you do not place stress on the knee or ankle joint. Below are different foot positions, based on a wall clock, to help you better understand exactly what the cues mean for each pose when foot placement is referenced to a number on the clock.

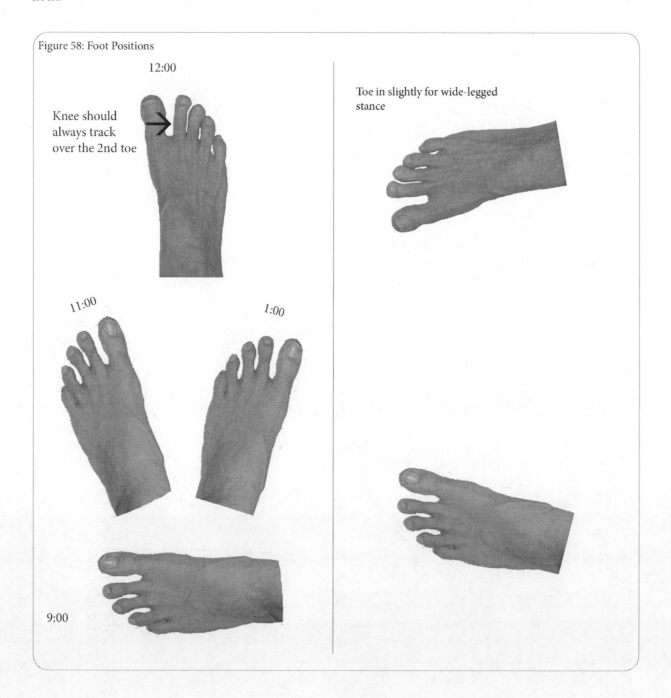

Figure 58: Foot Positions

# SEATED MEDITATION - SIDDHASANA

## Cues:

1. Fold a thick blanket or place a yoga pillow or block under your sit bones.

2. Place your feet together or cross your shins, widen your knees. If you cross your shins, slip each foot beneath the opposite knee. It is important to sit in a comfortable position as in figure 59.

3. Relax the feet so their outer edges rest comfortably on the floor.

4. As always, you should sit with your pelvis in a relatively neutral position by lengthening your tail bone and lifting your chest.

5. You can sit in this position for any length of time, but if you practice this pose regularly, be sure to alternate the cross of the legs. A good rule of thumb: On even-numbered days, cross the right shin in front of the left, and on odd-numbered days, do the opposite.

   Alternately, you can divide the practice time in half, and spend the first half with your right leg forward, and the second half with the left leg forward.

6. Keep your focus by practicing different breathing methods. You can draw the breath up the back of the spine for 6 counts, hold for 2 counts and exhale down the front of the body for 6 counts. Another method is to repeat a chant over and over as you inhale and exhale.

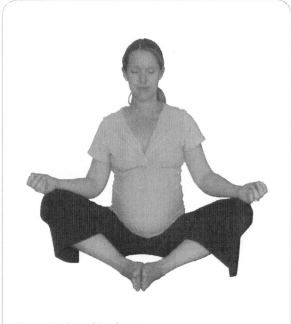

Figure 59: Seated Meditation

## Benefits:

1. Calms the brain.

2. Strengthens the back.

3. Stretches the knees and ankles.

# CAT AND COW

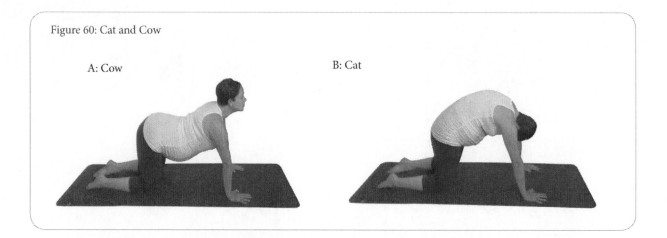

Figure 60: Cat and Cow

A: Cow          B: Cat

## Cues:

1. Start on your hands and knees in a "tabletop" position as in figure 61. Be sure your knees are directly below your hips and your wrists, elbows and shoulders are in line and perpendicular to the floor. Center your head in a neutral position, eyes looking at the floor.

2. As you inhale, lift your sit bones and chest toward the ceiling, allowing your belly to sink toward the floor slightly. Lift your head to look straight forward, figure 60A.

3. As you exhale, round the back like a "cat" drawing your belly button in lightly or if you are cramping, relax your belly letting your back muscles work, figure 60B.

4. Move slowly in and out of the pose, being careful not to over arch your back. If you feel any discomfort in the low back, bring the spine to neutral (table top figure 61) instead of the cow position.

## Benefits:

1. Pumps spinal fluid through the spine.

2. Opens up the upper and lower back.

3. Gentle massage to the internal organs.

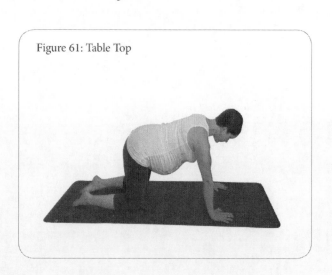

Figure 61: Table Top

## Precautions:

1. If you have a neck injury, keep the head in line with the torso.

2. When you are pregnant, this is the time to use your back muscles and let your abdominal muscles relax throughout the pose.

# SEATED BACK OPENER

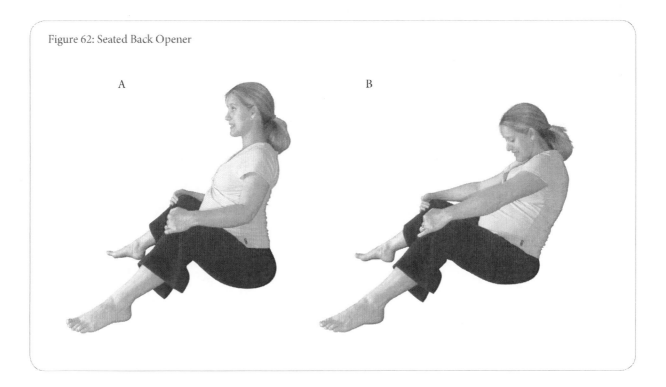

Figure 62: Seated Back Opener

A

B

## Cues:

1. Sit with your knees bent, feet outside your shoulders, grabbing your shins with your hands, pulling your chest up and lengthening your spine, and inhale, figure 62A. Keep eyes on the horizon.

2. Exhale and round your spine, supporting your back by holding onto your shins, figure 62B.

3. Repeat 5-10 times timed with breath.

## Benefits:

1. Pumps fluid into the pelvic and back area.

2. Stretches low back.

# COBBLER'S POSE - BADDHA KONASANA

## Cues:

1. Sit on the floor with the legs stretched out in front of you.

2. Bend the knees and bring the feet close to the trunk with the soles and heels of the feet together, figure 63.

3. Grab for the toes and open the feet so the outer sides of the feet pressed to the floor as you spread the feet wide.

4. Gaze straight ahead or down at your feet.

5. Hold for 5-10 breaths.

## Modifications:

1. Place the elbows on the thighs to increase stretch.

2. Exhale and bend forward, rest the head, then the nose and lastly the chin on the floor to increase stretch.

## Benefits:

1. Keeps the urinary bladder healthy.

2. Helps pregnant woman with delivery and reduces varicose veins (sit daily for a few minutes each day).

3. Stretches the groin and knees.

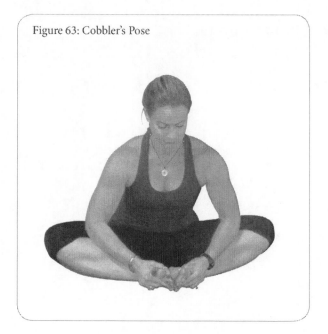

Figure 63: Cobbler's Pose

# SEATED GROIN, HAMSTRING AND BACK OPENER - MAHA MUDRA

## Cues:

1. Sit with legs apart, toes pointing toward the ceiling and bend the right leg.

2. Bring the left arm in front of the left leg, palm facing out, elbow against the knee

3. Reach the right arm over head, toward the right foot, figure 64.

4. Inhale as you reach up and exhale as you reach for the toes.

5. Repeat 5-10 times, timed with breath.

6. Switch sides.

## Modifications:

1. To deepen the stretch, reach for the toe as in figure 65A.

2. To deepen the back stretch reach the left hand to the right knee, as in figure 65B.

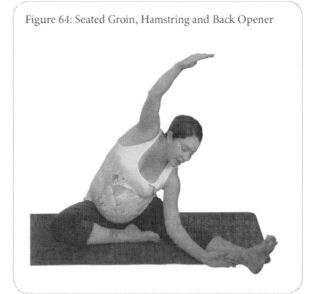

Figure 64: Seated Groin, Hamstring and Back Opener

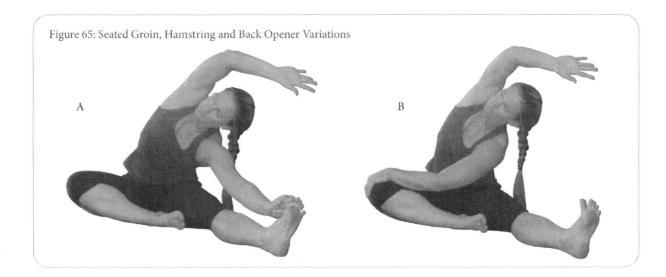

Figure 65: Seated Groin, Hamstring and Back Opener Variations

A

B

## Benefits:

1. Pumps fluid into the pelvic area and stretches the low back, quadratus lumborum, groin and hamstrings.

2. Tones the spleen and liver, thereby aiding in digestion.

# SEATED FORWARD FOLD - PASCHIMOTTANASANA

## Cues:

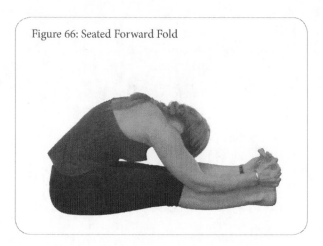

Figure 66: Seated Forward Fold

1. Sit with legs together and move the fleshy part of your bottom out of the way.

2. Bending from the hips, bring your torso toward your thighs. Exhale and try to grab the toes or simply place your hands on your thighs as in figure 66. Use a strap around your feet if you cannot reach your toes, but would like a deeper stretch.

3. Hold for 5-10 breaths.

4. As your belly grows, switch to seated splits below.

## Benefits:

1. Pumps fluid into the pelvic area and stretches the low back, groin, hamstrings, and quadratus lumborum.

2. Rejuvenates the spine and improves digestion.

3. A good stay in this pose massages the heart.

# SEATED SPLITS - UPAVISTHA KONASANA

## Cues:

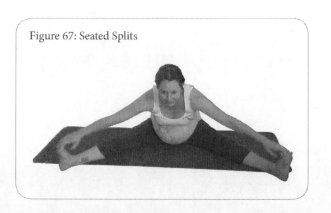

Figure 67: Seated Splits

1. Sit with legs spread apart as far as they can comfortably go with toes pointing toward the sky. Physically move your glutes and thigh out from under you to create space and allow your sit bones to make contact with the floor, figure 67.

2. Keeping your chest lifted, lean forward while grabbing your big toes, or placing your hands on your shins.

3 You can fold forward, placing your head on the floor or a block.

3. Hold this pose for 5 breaths.

## Benefits:

1. Stretches hamstrings and helps the blood to circulate in the pelvic region, thereby keeping it healthy.

# HAPPY BABY - ANANDA BALASANA

## Cues:

1. Lie on your back and grab the outside edges of your feet with your hands, figure 68.

2. Lengthen your tail bone and gently rock side to side for 5-10 breaths.

## Benefits:

1. Hip, groin and low back opener.

2. Relieves stress and emotions.

## Precautions:

1. If lying on your back causes you to feel dizzy or uncomfortable do not perform exercises on your back.

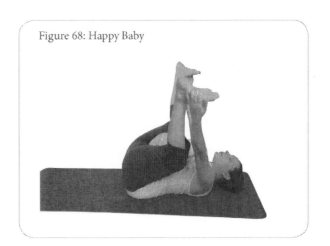
Figure 68: Happy Baby

# HIP EXTENSION - SETU BANDHA SARVANGASANA

## Cues:

1. Lie on your back, palms facing the ceiling, feet shoulder width apart and neck long by pressing the back of the head into the floor.

2. Start the movement by pressing your hips up using your buttocks, keeping the chest open and neck long, figure 69.

3. If it is comfortable, open your chest and clasp your hands under you to get a deeper stretch in the chest and shoulders.

4. Hold for 5-10 breaths.

## Benefits:

1. Hip, chest and shoulder opener.

2. Strengthens the buttocks and thighs.

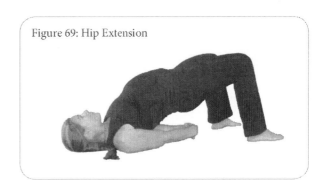
Figure 69: Hip Extension

## Precautions:

1. If you feel this in the low back, really squeeze your buttocks and lower the hips slightly.

2. If you feel pain in your neck, place a small rolled up towel under your neck.

# LEG ELEVATION - VIPARITA KARANI

## Cues:

1. Lie sideways against the wall and exhale as you swing your legs up onto the wall and lay your shoulders and head lightly down onto the floor, figure 70.

3. Lift and release the base of your skull away from the back of your neck and soften your throat (let your sternum lift toward the chin). Place a small roll (made from a hand towel for example) under your neck if the cervical spine feels flat. Open your shoulder blades away from the spine and release your hands and arms out to your sides, palms up.

4. Keep your legs relatively firm, just enough to hold them vertically in place. Release the heads of the thigh bones and the weight of your belly deeply into your torso, toward the back of the pelvis.

5. Stay in this pose anywhere from 5 to 15 minutes.

## Modifications:

1. This can also be done with the hands under the pelvis, or by placing a towel or block under the pelvis as in figure 71.

## Benefits:

1. Relieves tired or cramped legs and feet.

2. Gently stretches the back legs, front torso, and the back of the neck.

3. Relieves mild backache.

4. Calms the mind.

## Precautions:

1. If lying on your back causes you to feel dizzy or uncomfortable do not perform exercises on your back.

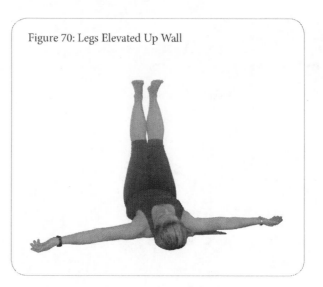

Figure 70: Legs Elevated Up Wall

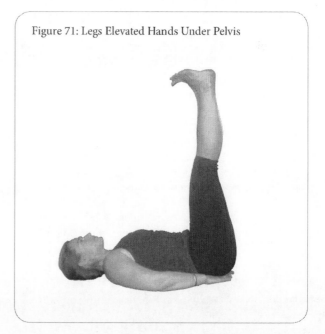

Figure 71: Legs Elevated Hands Under Pelvis

# BABY CRADLE

## Cues:

1. Sit with one leg extended and place the foot of the opposite leg in the crease of the elbow, figure 72.

2. Keep the chest lifted as you place the other arm outside the knee as if you were cradling a baby.

3. Gently rock side to side for 5-10 breaths.

4. Repeat on other side.

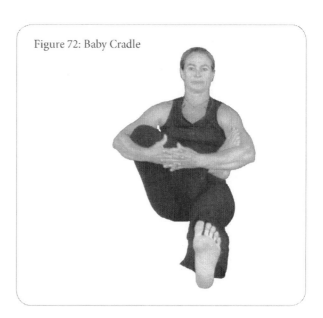

Figure 72: Baby Cradle

## Benefits:

1. Hip opener to relieve stress and emotions.

2. This will open your hips for pigeon.

## Precautions:

1. Avoid this pose if the hips feel too loose during the 3rd trimester.

# SEATED TWIST

## Cues:

1. Sit with your right knee bent and place it over your extended left leg, figure 73.

2. Keep eyes on the horizon, chest lifted and pull the bent leg toward the body.

3. Inhale and pull the leg closer, exhale and relax into the stretch.

4. Repeat 5-10 times, timed with breath.

5. Switch sides.

Figure 73: Seated Twist

## Benefits:

1. Opens the hips and releases emotions and stress.

## Modifications:

1. To make this stretch more advanced, bend the left leg, making sure both sit bones stay on the floor.

# SEATED PRETZEL - GOMUKHASANA

## Cues:

1. Sit in with both legs extended then bend your knees and put your feet on the floor.

2. Slide your right foot under the left knee to the outside of the left hip. Then cross your left leg over the right, stacking the left knee on top of the right and bring the left foot to the outside of the right hip.

3. Sit evenly on the sitting bones as in figure 74. If you are unable to keep both sit bones on the floor, keep the bottom leg extended.

4. Keep the chest lifted as you place your hands on your ankles and gently pull your legs toward you for a deeper stretch.

5. Hold for 5-10 breaths.

6. Repeat on other side.

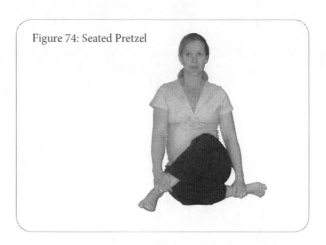

Figure 74: Seated Pretzel

## Precautions:

1. Avoid this pose if the hips feel too loose during the 3rd trimester.

## Benefits:

1. Hip opener to relieve stress and emotions.

2. This will open your hips for pigeon.

# SEATED GROIN AND HIP OPENER

## Cues:

1. Sit with one leg extended and grab the foot of the opposite leg, pulling the knee back so it is under your arm, figure 75.

2. Keep the chest lifted as you place the other arm on your thigh or on the floor for support.

3. Gently rock side to side for 5-10 breaths.

4. Repeat on other side.

## Benefits:

1. Hip opener to relieve stress and emotions.

2. This will open your hips for pigeon.

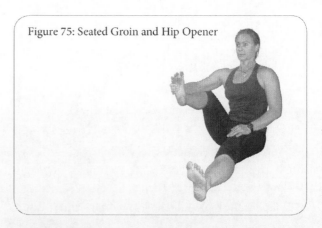

Figure 75: Seated Groin and Hip Opener

## Precautions:

1. Avoid this pose if the hips feel too loose during the 3rd trimester.

# THREAD THE NEEDLE - UPPER BODY

## Cues:

1. Kneel on the floor. Touch your big toes together and sit on your heels.

2. Reach your left arm under your body and look under your arm with your left ear on the floor.

3. Place your right palm on the floor, finger tips facing you and press into the floor to open the upper back, as in figure 76.

4. Hold this pose for 5 breaths.

5. Repeat on other side.

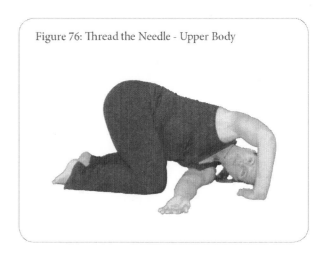

Figure 76: Thread the Needle - Upper Body

## Benefits:

1. Opens the thoracic spine and shoulders.

# THREAD THE NEEDLE - LOWER BODY

## Cues:

1. Lie on your back with knees bent. Place the right heel on the left upper thigh, figure 77.

2. For a deeper pose, lift the left foot off the floor and clasp your hands behind your left thigh.

3. Hold this pose for 5 breaths.

5. Repeat on other side.

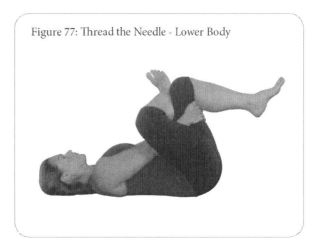

Figure 77: Thread the Needle - Lower Body

## Benefits:

1. Opens the hips and prepares the body for pigeon or can be done instead of pigeon.

## Precautions:

1. If lying on your back causes you to feel dizzy or uncomfortable do not perform exercises on your back.

## FIGURE 4

### Cues:

1. Lie on your back with knees bent and feet placed wider than your hips. Drop both knees to the right and place the right heel on the left thigh for a deeper stretch, figure 78.

2. Hold this pose for 5 breaths.

3. Repeat on other side.

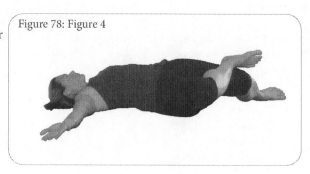
Figure 78: Figure 4

### Benefits:

1. Opens the hips and prepares the body for pigeon or can be done instead of pigeon.

2. Stretches the IT band (Iliotibial band).

## SPINAL ROTATION

### Cues:

1. Lie on your back with knees bent and feet placed wider than your hips.

2. Drop both knees to the left as in figure 79A and look right, keeping the shoulders on the floor.

3. Hold this pose for 5 breaths.

4. Repeat on other side.

### Modifications:

1. Place a yoga block between your knees if this bothers your low back, as in figure 79B.

### Precautions:

1. If you get light headed or dizzy with spinal rotations, do not do this pose.

### Benefits:

1. Opens the hips, reduces low back pain.

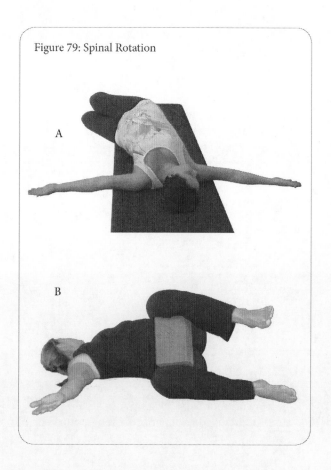
Figure 79: Spinal Rotation

A

B

# RECLINING BIG TOE POSE FOR HAMSTRINGS - SUPTA PADANGUSTHASANA

## Cues:

1. Lie on your back with knees bent and grab the right big toe with your hand or use a strap around the ball of the foot, as in figure 80.

2. Now straighten the left leg and pull the right leg toward you until you feel a comfortable stretch, making sure the right leg is straight. If the stretch is too strenuous, use the strap to lower the leg to a comfortable position.

3. Walk your hands up the strap until the elbows are fully extended. Broaden the shoulder blades across your back. Keeping the hands as high on the strap as possible, press the shoulder blades lightly into the floor as you open your chest.

4. Hold this pose for 5 breaths.

5. Now take the leg out to the side as in figure 81 and hold for 5 breaths.

6. Next, take the leg across the body as in figure 82 and hold for 5 breaths. If this bothers the low back, bend both knees.

7. Repeat this sequence on the left leg.

## Modifications:

1. If the stretch is too strenuous do not use the strap.

## Benefits:

1. Stretches hips, thighs, hamstrings, groins, and calves.

2. Strengthens the knees.

3. Improves digestion.

4. Relieves backache, sciatica, and menstrual discomfort.

5. Therapeutic for high blood pressure, flat feet, and infertility.

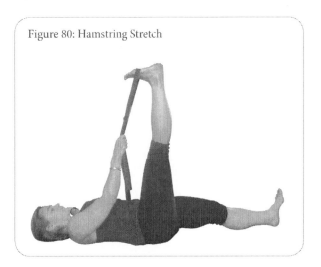

Figure 80: Hamstring Stretch

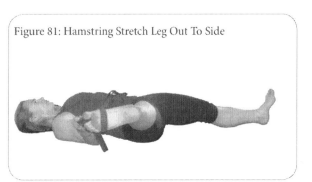

Figure 81: Hamstring Stretch Leg Out To Side

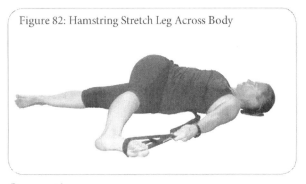

Figure 82: Hamstring Stretch Leg Across Body

## Precautions:

1. If lying on your back causes you to feel dizzy or uncomfortable do not perform exercises on your back.

# PIGEON - EKA PADA RAJAKAPOTASANA

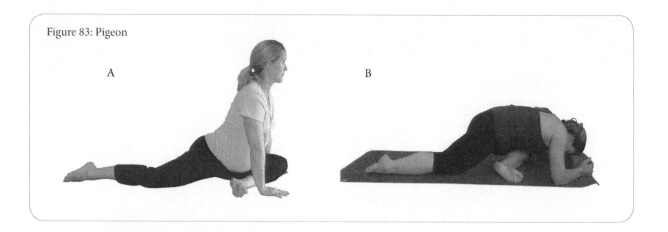

Figure 83: Pigeon

A

B

## Cues:

1. Begin on all fours.

2. Cross your left leg so that the bottom of your foot is against your right knee. Slowly lengthen your right leg straight behind you, keeping the top of the foot on the floor.

3. Align your hips so they are square as in figure 83A. Flex your left foot to protect your knee.

4. Place your hands beneath your shoulders and press into the floor. Lift your upper torso and raise your chest (think of a puffed-out pigeon chest) while keeping your shoulders down and away from the side of your head.

5. Hold for 3 to 5 breaths.

6. Uncross your left leg, straighten and shake it, then repeat on the other side.

## Modifications:

1. If this pose bothers your knee, be sure to flex your foot on the bent knee side and bring your shin closer to your body or place a pillow or block under the outside of your hip. You may also do the baby cradle instead on page 125, or thread the needle-lower body on page 127.

2. To get a deeper stretch in this pose, drape your upper body over the bent knee, placing your elbows on the ground and your head on a pillow, block or the floor, as in figure 83B.

## Benefits:

1. Opens up the hips and stretches the external rotators of the hips, allowing fluid movement during such exercises as a squat.

2. Relieves hip pain during the night if done before bed.

3. It can also help with urinary disorders.

# PIGEON WITH QUAD STRETCH

## Cues:

1. Begin on all fours.

2. Cross your left leg so that the bottom of your foot is against your right knee. Slowly lengthen your right leg straight behind you.

3. Align your hips so they are square, as in figure 83A.

4. Place your hands beneath your shoulders and press into the floor. Lift your upper torso and raise your chest (think of a puffed-out pigeon chest) while keeping your shoulders down and away from the side of your head.

5. If you feel balanced, reach back and grab the right foot behind to create a stretch in the front of the thigh, figure 84.

6. Hold for 3 to 5 breaths.

7. Release, straighten your legs and shake them, then repeat on the other side.

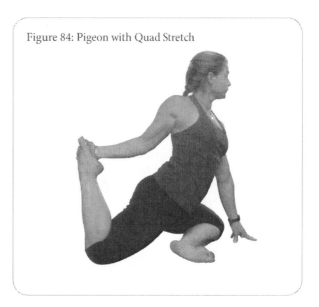

Figure 84: Pigeon with Quad Stretch

## Benefits:

1. Opens up the hips and stretches the external rotators of the hip and quadriceps (front of thigh), allowing fluid movement during such exercises as a squat.

2. Relieves hip pain during the night if done before bed.

3. It can also help with urinary disorders.

# CHILD'S POSE - BALASANA

## Cues:

1. Kneel on the floor. Touch your big toes together and sit on your heels, then separate your knees as wide as your hips, figure 85.

2. Exhale and lay your upper body between your thighs. Open across the back of your pelvis and lengthen your tailbone and gently place your forehead on the floor and relax your arms at your sides.

3. Hold this pose for 5 breaths or a few minutes.

## Modifications:

1. Place your head on a block or towel to support the neck.

2. Place the arms overhead as in figure 86 to lengthen the torso. Reach the arms long and without moving the arms, sit the buttocks back as far as you can.

## Benefits:

1. Calms the brain and helps relieve stress and mild depression.

2. Gently stretches the hips, thighs, and ankles.

3. Relieves back and neck pain when done with head and torso supported.

4. Should be done as a resting pose when the effort of your yoga practice has become too strenuous.

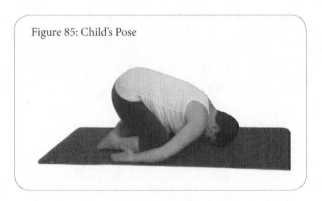

Figure 85: Child's Pose

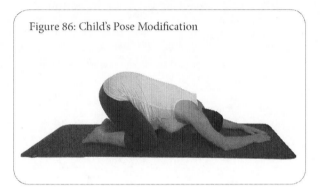

Figure 86: Child's Pose Modification

# DOWNWARD DOG

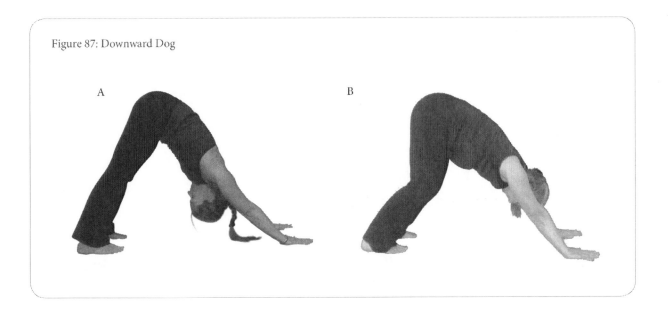

Figure 87: Downward Dog

A          B

## Cues:

1. Come onto the floor on your hands and knees. Set your knees directly below your hips and your hands slightly forward of your shoulders. Spread your fingers, gripping the mat and turn your toes under.

2. Exhale and lift your knees away from the floor, keeping the knees slightly bent and the heels lifted away from the floor, figure 87A. Lengthen your tailbone, pressing your hips up toward the ceiling. Lift the front of your thighs and activate the inner thigh.

3. Draw the belly button in slightly or simply just relax the belly if you feel any discomfort in the abdomen.

4. Open the shoulder blades by turning the palms out as if opening a jar. Relax the head and look toward your belly button.

5. If you cannot get the heels to the floor, bend your knees, as in figure 87B.

6. Hold this pose for 5 breaths.

## Benefits:

1. Calms the brain and helps relieve stress and mild depression

2. Energizes the body.

3. Stretches the shoulders, hamstrings, calves, arches, and hands and strengthens the arms and legs.

4. Helps prevent osteoporosis.

5. Improves digestion, relieves headaches, insomnia, back pain, and fatigue.

6. Therapeutic for high blood pressure, asthma, flat feet, sciatica, and sinusitis.

# PLANK

## Cues:

1. From a downward dog position, pull your chest forward, keeping your wrists under your shoulders, gripping the mat with your fingers.

2. Squeeze your shoulder blades together and lengthen your spine, keeping your hips in line with your shoulders. A good plank position is when your sacrum, shoulders and head are in one line as shown in figure 88, with a dowel rod on your back as a feedback mechanism.

3  Glutes and thighs are contracted, belly button drawn in lightly or not at all. You may use your back muscles to maintain good form.

4. Hold for 5 breaths or 20-60 seconds.

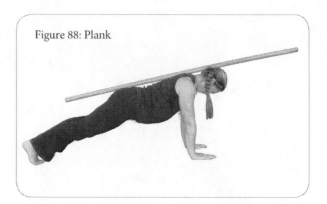

Figure 88: Plank

## Modifications:

1. To make this exercise easier, drop your knees to the floor. This exercise should only be done as a transitional pose in a sequence. In the third trimester, avoid this pose and perform a table top pose instead.

## Benefits:

1. Strengthens the upper body and core.

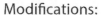

# INDIAN SQUAT

## Cues:

1. Begin by standing with your feet a little more than shoulder width apart. Exhale and squat down letting your spine round (let the heels come up if they have to). You can place a block under your buttocks if it is hard to get into the squat position.

2. Place your hands in prayer position over the sternum and press the thighs apart with the outside of your arms, as in figure 89.

3. Be sure to keep your chest lifted and eyes on the horizon.

4. Hold for 5 breaths or 20-60 seconds.

## Modifications:

1. To make this exercise easier, hold onto something firm, like a table, to help you find stability while you learn to press your heels down and lengthen your spine. This variation will also help you stretch your calves and ankles so that you can reach your heels to the floor. The object you hold onto should be fixed, secure, and high enough so that your arms can reach upward in the squat.

## Benefits:

1. The squat position stretches the ankles, groin and back. This also takes a great deal of pressure off the spine during pregnancy.

2. Tones the belly.

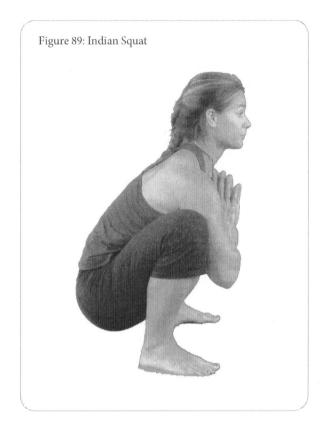

Figure 89: Indian Squat

# MOUNTAIN POSE - TADASANA

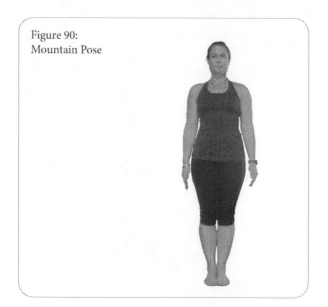

Figure 90:
Mountain Pose

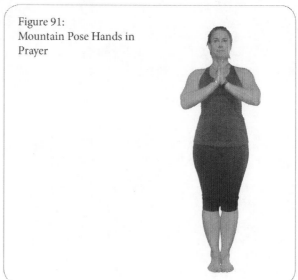

Figure 91:
Mountain Pose Hands in
Prayer

## Cues:

1. Stand tall with feet together, heels and big toes touching. Press all 10 toes into the floor, distributing the weight of your body evenly as in figure 90.

2. Lift the knee caps, rotating the inner thighs toward midline. Then, imagine a string pulling you up from the crown of your head. Lengthen your tailbone toward the floor and lift the pubis toward the belly button.

3. Squeeze your shoulder blades together, then widen them across the back. Lift your chest and hang your arms beside the torso.

4. Balance the crown of your head directly over the center of your pelvis, with the underside of your chin parallel to the floor, throat soft, and the tongue wide and flat on the floor of your mouth. Soften your eyes.

5. Tadasana is usually the starting position for all the standing poses, but it's useful to practice Tadasana as a pose in itself. Stay in the pose for 30 seconds to 1 minute, breathing easily.

## Modifications:

1. Bring hands to prayer to center yourself, thumbs pressing into the sternum, as in figure 91.

## Benefits:

1. Improves posture.

2. Strengthens thighs, knees, and ankles.

3. Firms abdomen and buttocks.

4. Relieves sciatica.

5. Reduces flat feet.

## UPWARD SALUTE - URDHVA HASTASANA

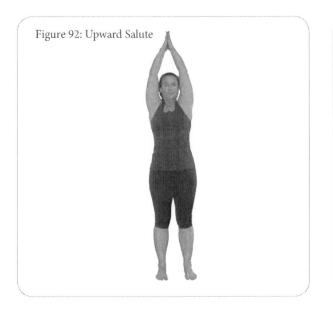

Figure 92: Upward Salute

## STANDING FORWARD BEND - UTTANASANA

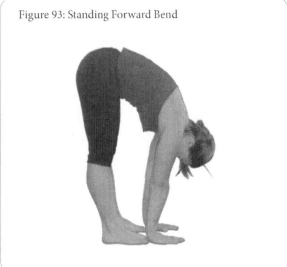

Figure 93: Standing Forward Bend

## Cues:

1. Stand as you would in mountain pose and reach your heart and arms up to the sun. If it is difficult to keep the feet together, place them shoulder width apart, as in figure 92.

2. At the peak of the pose, the arms converge over your head as you bring your palms together. Spread your shoulder blades and draw your chin in slightly (towards the center of the throat), as you take your head back and gaze at your thumbs. If you have neck issues, gaze forward, eyes on the horizon.

3. Hold for 5 breaths or one minute.

## Benefits:

1. Stretches the belly.

2. Improves digestion.

3. Stretches the shoulders and armpits.

4. Helps relieve mild anxiety.

## Cues:

1. Stand in mountain pose, hands on hips. Exhale and bend forward from the hip joints, not from the waist, as in figure 93. As you descend, lift the knee caps and turn the inner thighs back.

2. Continue to lengthen through the torso and the backs of the legs as you place your hands on the thighs or floor. You can also grab the elbows and hang.

3. Hold for 5 breaths.

## Benefits:

1. Calms the brain and helps relieve stress.

2. Stimulates the liver and kidneys.

3. Stretches the hamstrings, calves, and hips.

4. Strengthens the thighs and knees.

5. Improves digestion.

6. Reduces fatigue and anxiety.

7. Relieves headaches and insomnia.

8. Therapeutic for asthma, high blood pressure, infertility, osteoporosis, and sinusitis.

## STANDING FORWARD BEND GRABBING BIG TOES - PADANGUSTHASANA

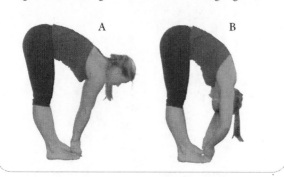

Figure 94: Standing Forward Bend Grabbing Big Toes

A          B

### Cues:

1. Stand in mountain pose, hands on hips. Exhale and bend forward from the hip joints, not from the waist. As you descend lift the knee caps and turn the inner thighs back.

2. Continue to lengthen through the torso and the backs of the legs.

3. Grab the big toe on each foot with your index and middle fingers (peace fingers), figure 94A.

4. Use your biceps to pull your torso closer to your thighs, elbows coming out and then relax and lengthen through the spine, figure 94B. Bend knees if needed.

5. Repeat for 5 breaths.

### Benefits:

1. Calms the brain and helps relieve stress.

2. Stimulates the liver and kidneys.

3. Stretches the hamstrings, calves, and hips.

4. Strengthens the thighs and knees.

5. Improves digestion.

6. Reduces fatigue and anxiety.

7. Relieves headaches and insomnia.

8. Therapeutic for asthma, high blood pressure, infertility, osteoporosis, and sinusitis.

## HALF STANDING FORWARD BEND

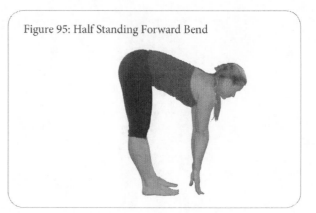

Figure 95: Half Standing Forward Bend

### Cues:

1. Stand in mountain pose, hands on hips. Exhale and bend forward from the hip joints, not from the waist. As you descend, lift the knee caps and turn the inner thighs back.

2. Continue to lengthen through the torso and the backs of the legs.

3. Inhale and lengthen your spine, gaze is lifted, and the spine is extended while the fingertips stay on the floor or rise to the shins, figure 95.

4. Repeat for 5 breaths.

### Benefits:

1. Calms the brain and helps relieve stress.

2. Stimulates the liver and kidneys.

3. Stretches the hamstrings, calves, and hips.

4. Strengthens the thighs and knees.

5. Improves digestion.

6. Reduces fatigue and anxiety.

7. Relieves headaches and insomnia.

8. Therapeutic for asthma, high blood pressure, infertility, osteoporosis, and sinusitis.

# STANDING SQUAT - UTKATASANA

## Cues:

1. Stand in Mountain Pose (Tadasana). Inhale and raise your arms overhead, arms near ears. Either keep the arms parallel, palms facing inward, or join the palms.

2. Exhale and bend your knees, trying to take the thighs as nearly parallel to the floor as possible without letting the knees pass the toes, as in figure 96.

3. The torso will lean slightly forward over the thighs until the front torso forms approximately a right angle with the tops of the thighs.

4. Keep the inner thighs parallel to each other.

5. Firm your shoulder blades against the back.

6. Take your tailbone down toward the floor and in toward your pubis to keep the lower back long.

7. Stay for 30 seconds to a minute.

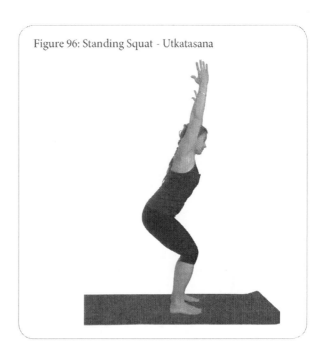

Figure 96: Standing Squat - Utkatasana

## Modifications:

1. The traditional yoga pose requires the knees to come forward over the toes to increase intensity. Only perform the pose this way if you have no previous knee injuries and do not feel any knee pain.

## Benefits:

1. Strengthens the ankles, thighs, calves, and spine.

2. Stretches shoulders and chest.

3. Stimulates the abdominal organs, diaphragm, and heart.

4. Reduces flat feet.

# STANDING BACK BEND

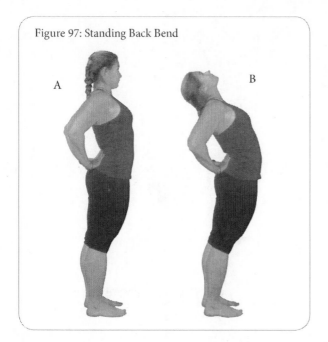

Figure 97: Standing Back Bend

A    B

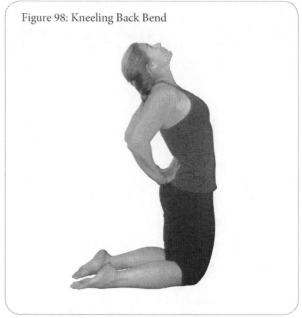

Figure 98: Kneeling Back Bend

## Cues:

1. Stand tall with feet together, heels and big toes touching. Press all 10 toes into the floor, distributing the weight of your body evenly.

2. Place the hands on the low back, with the fingers toward the head, figure 97A.

3. Squeeze your shoulder blades together, then widen them across the back and release them down your back. Lift your chest.

4. Squeeze your buttocks and gently extend back, as in figure 97B.

5. Stay in the pose for 15 seconds to 1 minute, breathing easily.

## Modifications:

1. This can also be done kneeling as in figure 98, with a blanket or a mat folded up under your knees for support.

## Benefits:

1. Improves posture.

2. Strengthens thighs, back, knees, and ankles.

3. Firms abdomen and buttocks.

4. Relieves sciatica.

5. Reduces flat feet.

6. Stretches chest, abdomen and low back.

# STANDING WIDE-LEGGED FORWARD BEND - PRASARITA PADOTTANASANA

## Cues:

1. Stand in mountain pose, hands on hips and jump or walk your feet 4-5 feet apart, depending on your flexibility. Make sure your feet are slightly pigeon toed, as in figure 99A.

2. Exhale and bend forward from the hip joints, not from the waist, with airplane arms, as in figure 99B.

3. As you descend, tighten the legs by drawing up on your knee caps.

4. Continue to lengthen through the torso and the backs of the legs and place your palms on the floor in line with your shoulders, figure 99C.

5. Hold for 5 breaths.

## Modifications:

1. If this pose places too much stress on the hamstrings (back of thighs), then bring the legs closer together.

2. To decrease stress on the neck, simply hold your elbows and let your head hang.

3. You may increase intensity and open the shoulders by interlacing the fingers and letting your arms come over the head, as in figure 99D. If this is difficult, but you would like to open the chest, simply grab the elbows behind you.

## Benefits:

1. Strengthens and stretches the inner thighs, back of the legs and the spine.

2. Tones the abdominal organs.

3. Calms the brain and releases neck tension.

4. Relieves mild backache and helps to relax neck.

5. Releases emotions.

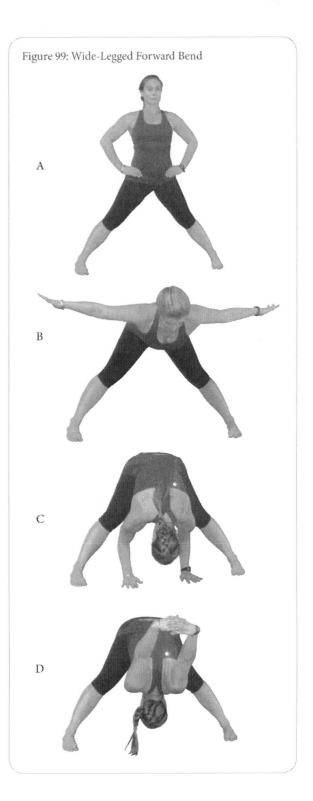

Figure 99: Wide-Legged Forward Bend

A

B

C

D

# STANDING WIDE-LEGGED FORWARD BEND WITH TWIST - PRASARITA PADOTTANASANA

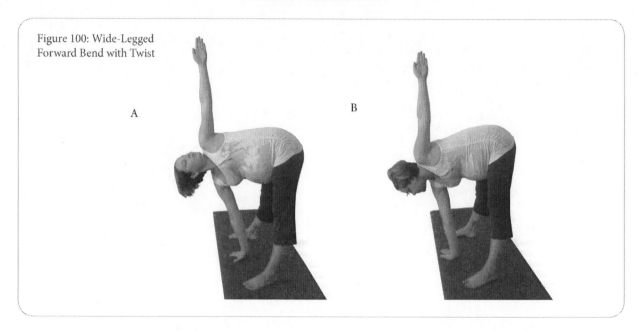

Figure 100: Wide-Legged Forward Bend with Twist

A

B

## Cues:

1. Stand in mountain pose, hands on hips and walk your feet 4-5 feet apart, depending on your flexibility. Make sure your feet are slightly pigeon toed.

2. Exhale and bend forward from the hip joints, not from the waist. As you descend, tighten the legs by drawing up on your knee caps.

3. Continue to lengthen through the torso and the backs of the legs and place your right palm on the floor, in line with your shoulder or slightly forward, finger tips facing forward or to the right, figure 100A.

4. Extend the left arm straight up, palm facing left and look up toward the left thumb.

5. Hold for 5 breaths and switch sides.

## Modifications:

1. If this pose places too much stress on the hamstrings (back of thighs) then bring the legs closer together.

2. To decrease stress on the neck, look toward the floor as in figure 100B.

## Benefits:

1. Strengthens and stretches the inner thighs, back of the legs and the spine.

2. Tones the abdominal organs.

3. Calms the brain and releases neck tension.

4. Relieves mild backache and helps to relax neck.

5. Releases emotions.

# TREE POSE - VRKSASANA ONE

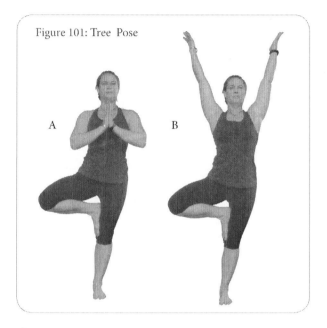

Figure 101: Tree Pose

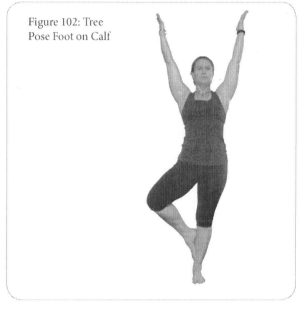

Figure 102: Tree
Pose Foot on Calf

## Cues:

1. Stand in mountain pose and shift your weight slightly onto the left foot, keeping the inner foot and big toe ball mount planted on the floor.

2. Draw your right foot up and place the heel against the inner left thigh, above the knee joint and press the right heel into the inner left groin, toes pointing toward the floor, as in figure 101A.

3. The center of your pelvis should be directly over the left foot.

4. Rest your hands on the top rim of your pelvis. Make sure the pelvis is in a neutral position, with the top rim parallel to the floor.

5. Lengthen your tailbone toward the floor. Firmly press the right foot sole against the inner thigh and resist with the outer left leg. Press your hands together in prayer and gaze softly at a fixed point in front of you. Once you have your balance, raise the arms up like the branches of a tree, as in figure 101B.

6. Hold for 5 breathes or one minute.

7. Repeat on other side.

## Modifications:

1. If your balance has not developed to the point you can stand on one foot easily, stand near a wall for support.

2. If you cannot place your right foot above your knee simply place it on your calf, below the knee joint, as in figure 102.

3. To decrease the intensity, simply leave your hands in prayer position.

4. To increase the intensity, look up toward the ceiling, tongue on the roof of the mouth.

## Benefits:

1. Improves posture and balance.

2. Strengthens thighs, knees, and ankles.

3. Firms abdomen and buttocks.

4. Relieves sciatica.

5. Reduces flat feet.

# WARRIOR I

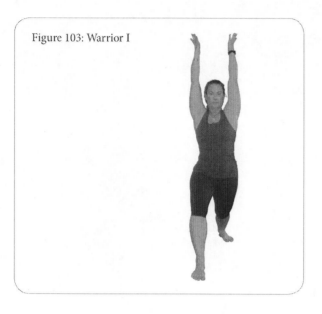

Figure 103: Warrior I

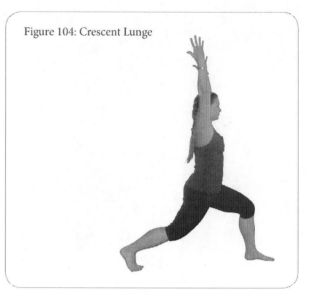

Figure 104: Crescent Lunge

## Cues:

1. From standing, feet shoulder width apart, with your hands on your hips, step your left foot back 3-4 feet and angle your left foot to about 11:00 (30 degrees). Keep your right foot pointing forward. With your left heel firmly anchored to the floor and the outer edge of the foot connecting to the mat, exhale and bend your right knee over the right ankle so the shin is perpendicular to the floor, as in figure 103. Keep your hips square to the front of the mat.

2. Raise your arms and reach actively through the little-finger sides of the hands toward the ceiling. Squeeze your shoulder blades together and relax your shoulders away from your ears.

3. Reach strongly through your arms, opening your heart. As you press the back foot into the mat, reach for the ceiling, and if possible, bring the palms together.

4. Keep your head in a neutral position, gazing forward, or tilt it back and look up at your hands.

5. Hold for 5 breaths or 1 minute.

6. Repeat on other side.

## Modifications:

1. If your knee bothers you on the back leg, lift the heel and turn the toes so they face forward, as with a crescent lunge, figure 104.

2. To increase the intensity bend the front leg more.

3. To decrease the intensity, bring the hands to the hips.

## Benefits:

1. Stretches the chest, lungs, shoulders, neck, belly, groin and hip flexors.

2. Strengthens the shoulders and arms, and the muscles of the back.

3. Strengthens and stretches the thighs, calves, and ankles.

# WARRIOR II - VIRABHADRASANA II

## Cues:

1. From standing with your hands on your hips, step your left foot back and angle your left foot to about 9:00 so the outer edge of your foot is in line with the short edge of the mat. Keep your right foot pointing forward and bend your right leg, getting as close to parallel to the floor as possible, keeping your knee over the ankle with the right shin perpendicular to the floor, as in figure 105.

2. With the left outer edge of your foot connecting to the mat, open your hips so they are square with the long edge of the mat and contract your thigh muscles as you tuck the tail bone under.

3. Raise your arms out to the side, so they are parallel to the floor, palms facing the floor. Squeeze your shoulder blades together and relax your shoulders away from your ears.

4. Keep your head in a neutral position, gazing out over your right middle finger.

5. Hold for 5 breaths or 1 minute.

6. Repeat on other side.

## Modifications:

1. Only go as low into the lunge as your body will comfortably allow.

2. To increase the intensity, bend the front leg more placing the right forearm on the right leg, and reach the left hand over the head, reaching through the pinky finger as in figure 106, Extended Side Angle Pose on page 146.

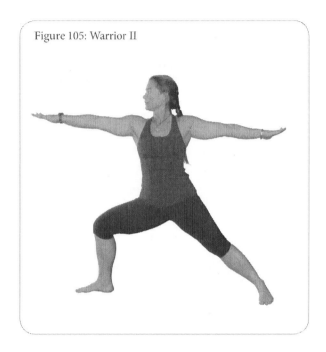

Figure 105: Warrior II

## Benefits:

1. Strengthens and stretches the legs and ankles.

2. Stretches groin, chest, lungs, and shoulders.

3. Stimulates abdominal organs.

4. Increases stamina.

5. Relieves backaches, especially through second trimester of pregnancy.

6. Therapeutic for carpal tunnel syndrome, flat feet, infertility, osteoporosis, and sciatica and ankles.

# EXTENDED SIDE ANGLE - UTTHITA PARSVAKONASANA

## Cues:

1. From standing with your hands on your hips, step your left foot back and angle your left foot to about 9:00 so the outer edge of your foot is in line with the short edge of the mat. Keep your right foot pointing forward and bend your right leg, getting as close to parallel to the floor as possible, keeping your knee over the ankle, with the right shin perpendicular to the floor.

2. With the left outer edge of your foot connecting to the mat, open your hips so they are square with the long edge of the mat and contract your thigh muscles as you tuck the tail bone under.

3. Raise your arms out to the side, so they are parallel to the floor, palms facing the floor. Squeeze your shoulder blades together and relax your shoulders away from your ears.

4. Place your right forearm on the right leg and reach the left hand over, extending the left side long, as in figure 106.

5. Hold for 5 breaths or 1 minute.

6. Repeat on other side.

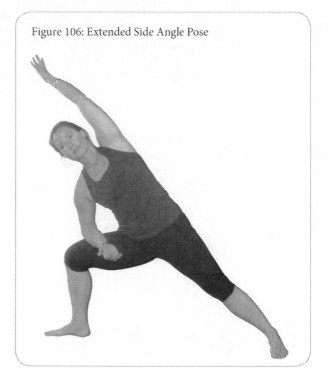

Figure 106: Extended Side Angle Pose

## Modifications:

1. If it bothers your neck to gaze at your hand, then simply gaze straight ahead.

## Benefits:

1. Strengthens and stretches the legs, knees, and ankles.

2. Stretches the groin, spine, waist, chest, lungs, and shoulders.

3. Stimulates abdominal organs.

4. Increases stamina.

# TRIANGLE - TRIKONASANA

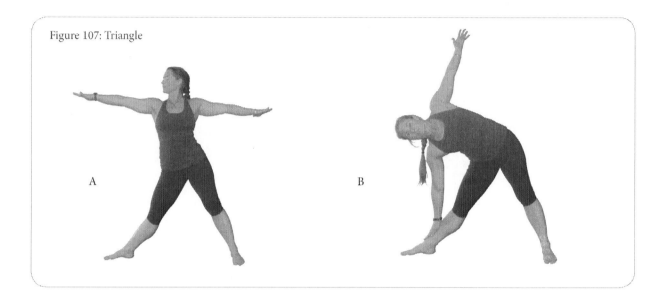

Figure 107: Triangle

A

B

## Cues:

1. From standing, with your hands on your hips, step your left foot back and angle your left foot to about 9:00, so the outer edge of your foot is in line with the mat. Keep your right foot pointing forward and right leg straight.

2. With the left outer edge of your foot connecting to the mat, open your hips so they are square with the long edge of the mat and contract your thigh muscles.

3. Raise your arms out to the side, so they are parallel to the floor, palms facing the floor. Squeeze your shoulder blades together and relax your shoulders away from your ears, figure 107A.

4. Reach your right hand and torso to the right as far as you can go and then side bend placing your hand on top of your foot or on the floor near the right foot.

5. Turn the left foot slightly to the right, keeping the left leg stretched from the inside and tightened at the knee, figure 107B.

6. Stretch the left arm up, bringing it in line with the right shoulder and extend the trunk, with a jazz hand (fingers spread wide). Keep the chest open and lifted.

7. If it is comfortable, gaze up at the left thumb.

8. Hold for 5 breaths or 1 minute.

9. Repeat on other side.

## Modifications:

1. Use a block or blocks under your hand if the stretch is too much. It is important to keep the legs straight to get the most out of this pose.

## Benefits:

1. Strengthens and stretches the legs, hips and ankles.

2. Relieves back and neck sprains.

3. Develops the chest.

# SIDE LYING SAVASANA

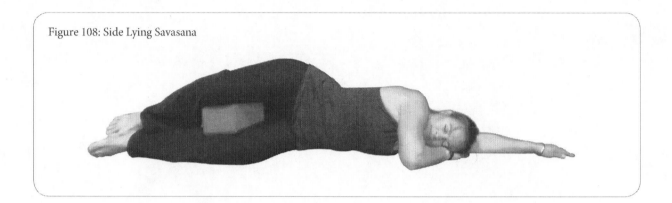

Figure 108: Side Lying Savasana

## Cues:

1. During pregnancy, it's essential that the body be placed in a side-lying position. Lie on your left side, on a mat or blanket with head and legs supported with a bolster or blanket, as in figure 108.

2. Stretch your arms over head, tighten your thighs and face, and then release everything with a deep sigh.

3. Cover with a blanket to keep warm.

4. Start by relaxing the breath and bringing your focus inward, clearing your mind of all thoughts and to do lists. If a thought comes into your mind say "that's a nice thought, now go away."

5. Hold for 5-10 minutes.

## Benefits:

1. Calms the brain and helps relieve stress and mild depression.

2. Relaxes the body.

3. Reduces headaches, fatigue, and insomnia.

4. Helps to lower blood pressure.

## QUIZ #4

1.    Which part of the body holds emotions?

    _____

2.    Name 3 poses to reduce sciatic nerve pain?

    _____, _____, _____

3.    Which pose is optimal for preparing for labor?

    _____

4.    Which toe should the knee track over duing standing poses?

    _____

5.    Which poses help calm the mind?

    _____

# PRENATAL YOGA SEQUENCES

The following yoga sequences are ideal for pregnant women. Choose the yoga sequence based on your level of ability and comfort. The sequences are in order of the least challenging to the most challenging. Each yoga sequence is about 3-5 minutes in length. If your goal is to perform your yoga sequences for 30 minutes, simply repeat the same sequence over and over, or combine some of your favorite yoga sequences together. For example you can warm up with the low energy sequence and then follow it with sun salutation A and finish with hip opener.

Remember, detailed instructions for each pose can be found in the yoga chapter. The page number for each pose is listed in the yoga sequence table, just above the picture.

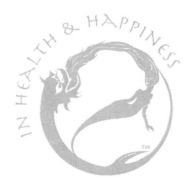

IN HEALTH & HAPPINESS

# LOW ENERGY SEQUENCE

## PRENATAL SEQUENCE - LOW ENERGY

This sequence is excellent for those who are on reduced activity, are feeling very sick and sluggish and simply do not have energy during the day.

| Exercise | Description | Breaths | Notes |
|---|---|---|---|
| Seated Meditation page 117 | Sit quietly in a comfortable position on the floor or elevate the hips with a block or blanket. | 10 breaths, inhaling up the spine for 6 counts, hold for 2 counts at the top and exhaling down the spine for 6 counts. | |
| Cat Pose page 118 | Come to all fours and round the back like a cat as you exhale. | 1-5 breaths | |
| Cow Pose page 118 | Inhale and release the back like a cow. If this places stress on the low back, come to table top pose shown in the notes section. | 1-5 breaths | Table Top page 118 |
| Thread The Needle - Upper Body page 127 | Slide the left hand under the body and place the right palm by the face, with the elbow bent. Press the right palm into the floor and rotate, opening the shoulder. | 1-5 breaths and then switch sides | |
| Thread The Needle - Lower Body page127 | Lie on your back with knees bent and bring your right foot on top your left thigh. If you need more stretch pull the left leg toward the body. | 1-5 breaths and then switch sides | |

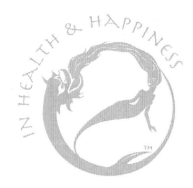

IN HEALTH & HAPPINESS

# PRENATAL YOGA SEQUENCE - LOW BACK PAIN SEATED

# PRENATAL YOGA SEQUENCE - LOW BACK PAIN SEATED

This sequence is excellent for anytime you have low back pain and can be done right before bed and right when you wake up.

| Exercise | Description | Breaths | Notes |
|---|---|---|---|
| Seated Meditation page 117 | Sit quietly in a comfortable position on the floor or elevate the hips with a block or blanket. | 10 breaths, inhaling up the spine for 6 counts, hold for 2 counts at the top and exhaling down the spine for 6 counts. | |
| Cat Pose page 118 | Come to all fours and round the back like a cat as you exhale. | 1-5 breaths | |
| Cow Pose page 118 | Inhale and release the back like a cow. If this places stress on the low back, come to table top pose shown in the notes section. | 1-5 breaths | Table Top page 118 |
| Seated Back Opener page 119 | Sit tall and bend your knees grabbing the tops of your shins with your hands. Inhale and pull your chest forward. | 1-5 breaths | |
| Seated Back Opener page 119 | Sit tall and bend your knees grabbing the tops of your shins with your hands. Exhale and round your back. | 1-5 breaths | |

# PRENATAL YOGA SEQUENCE - LOW BACK PAIN SEATED CONTINUED

This sequence is excellent for anytime you have low back pain and can be done right before bed and right when you wake up.

| Exercise | Description | Breaths | Notes |
|---|---|---|---|
| Child Pose<br>page 132 | Fold forward, with feet together and knees wide, to allow a place for your belly to drop. Extend you hands over head or place them by your sides. | 5-10 breaths | |
| Seated Hamstring and Low Back Opener<br>page 121 | Sit with your left leg extended, toes pointing up, and reach your left arm inside the left leg opening your chest and then reach the right arm over. | 5-10 breaths | |
| Seated Splits<br>page 122 | Sit with your legs apart, as wide as you can comfortably go, with toes pointing up. Lean forward and grab your toes or place your forearms on the floor. | 5-10 breaths | |
| Seated Hamstring and Low Back Opener<br>page 121 | Sit with your right leg extended, toes pointing up, and reach your right arm inside the right leg, opening your chest, and then reach the left arm over. | 5-10 breaths | |
| Indian Squat<br>page 135 | Come to your feet with the feet wider than shoulder width. Place your hands in prayer, elbows inside the knees and bring your thumbs to your sternum. | 5-10 breaths | Sit on a block if you cannot get the heels to the floor. |

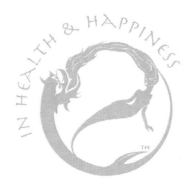

# PRENATAL YOGA SEQUENCE - LOW BACK PAIN STANDING

# PRENATAL YOGA SEQUENCE - LOW BACK PAIN STANDING

This sequence is excellent for anytime you have low back pain and cannot be seated.

| Exercise | Description | Breaths | Notes |
|---|---|---|---|
| Standing Back Extension page 140 | Stand with palms on your back, finger tips facing toward your head. Squeeze your buttocks and gently push forward. | 5-10 breaths. Modify by coming to your knees with a blanket under your knees. | |
| Standing Wide-legged Forward Bend page 141 | Take your legs wider than shoulder width, toes slightly in and fold forward, lifting the knee caps. | 5-10 breaths | |
| Standing Wide-legged Forward-Bend with Twist page 142 | From the position above, place the right hand on the floor and rotate to the left. | 5-10 breaths | |
| Standing Wide-legged Forward Bend with Twist page 142 | From the position above, place the left hand on the floor and rotate to the right. | 5-10 breaths | |
| Leg Elevation Up Wall page 124 | End this sequence with your legs placed up a wall. Make sure you get your buttocks close to the wall first, then extend the legs. | 1-5 minutes | |

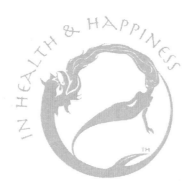

# LIVER, DIGESTION & BLADDER STANDING SEQUENCE

# LIVER, DIGESTION AND BLADDER STANDING SEQUENCE

This sequence is excellent for anytime you have digestive issues or frequent urination.

| Exercise | Description | Breaths | Notes |
|---|---|---|---|
| Mountain Pose page 136 | Stand with hands in prayer, feet together. | Hold for one breath | |
| Standing Wide-legged Forward Bend page 141 | Walk your feet 4-5 feet apart, with the toes turned slightly inward, hands on the hips. | One breath | |
| Standing Wide-legged Forward Bend page 141 | Exhale and fold halfway, with the arms out to the side, lifting the knee caps and hold. | 1-5 breaths | |
| Standing Wide-legged Forward Bend page 141 | Fold all the way forward, placing the palms on the floor or blocks. | 5-10 breaths | |

# LIVER, DIGESTION AND BLADDER STANDING SEQUENCE CONTINUED

This sequence is excellent for anytime you have digestive issues or frequent urination.

| Exercise | Description | Breaths | Notes |
|----------|-------------|---------|-------|
| Standing Wide-legged Forward Bend with Twist page 142 | Place the right hand on the floor and rotate to the left lifting the left arm up. | 5-10 breaths and switch sides | |
| Standing Wide-legged Forward Bend page 141 | Place your hands on your hips. slightly bend your knees and return to standing | 1-5 breaths | |
| Mountain Pose page 136 | Bring your feet together with hands in prayer. | 1-5 breaths | |

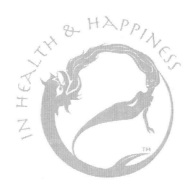

IN HEALTH & HAPPINESS

# LIVER, DIGESTION, BLADDER SEATED SEQUENCE

# LIVER, DIGESTION AND BLADDER SEATED SEQUENCE

This sequence is excellent for anytime you have digestive issues or frequent urination.

| Exercise | Description | Breaths | Notes |
|---|---|---|---|
| Cobbler's Pose page 120 | Sit quietly, placing the feet together and open up your toes as you press your thighs down with your elbows. | 10 breaths inhaling up the spine for 6 counts, hold for 2 counts at the top and exhaling down the spine for 6 counts. | |
| Seated Hamstring and Low Back Opener page 121 | Sit with your left leg extended, toes pointing up, and reach your left arm inside the left leg, opening your chest and then reach the right arm over. | 5-10 breaths and then switch sides | |
| Seated Forward Fold page 122 | Bring both legs together and round your back as you reach for your toes or rest your forearms on your thighs. | 5-10 breaths | Perform seated splits when the belly becomes too large.<br><br>Seated Splits page 122 |
| Seated Pretzel page 126 | Sit tall, placing your left leg over the right and bring the right heel toward the body if it is comfortable. Pull the left leg toward you. | 5-10 breaths and then switch sides | |

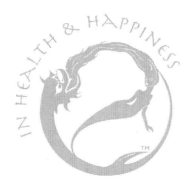

# PRENATAL YOGA SEQUENCE - LABOR

## PRENATAL YOGA SEQUENCE - LABOR

This sequence helps prepare you for labor and can be done frequently as you get closer to your due date.

| Exercise | Description | Breaths | Notes |
|---|---|---|---|
| Cobbler's Pose page 120 | Sit quietly, placing the feet together and open up your toes as you press your thighs down with your elbows. | 10 breaths inhaling up the spine for 6 counts, hold for 2 counts at the top and exhaling down the spine for 6 counts. | |
| Cat Pose page 118 | Come to all fours and round the back like a cat as you exhale. | 1-5 breaths | |
| Cow Pose page 118 | Inhale and release the back like a cow. If this places stress on the low back, come to table top pose shown in the notes section. | 1-5 breaths | Table Top page 118 |
| Seated Back Opener page 119 | Sit tall and bend your knees grabbing the tops of your shins with your hands. Inhale and pull your chest forward. | 1-5 breaths | |
| Seated Back Opener page 119 | Sit tall and bend your knees, grabbing the tops of your shins with your hands. Exhale and round your back. | 1-5 breaths | |

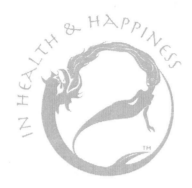

IN HEALTH & HAPPINESS

# HIP OPENER

# PRENATAL YOGA SEQUENCE - HIP OPENER

This sequence is excellent for opening the hips and releasing emotional issues and can be done right before bed and right when you wake up.

| Exercise | Description | Breaths | Notes |
|---|---|---|---|
| Cobbler's Pose page 120 | Sit quietly, placing the feet together and open up your toes as you press your thighs down with your elbows. | 10 breaths inhaling up the spine for 6 counts, hold for 2 counts at the top and exhaling down the spine for 6 counts. | |
| Baby Cradle page 125 | Extend your left leg and cradle your right leg like a baby, keeping your chest lifted. Switch sides. This can be done on your back if it is easier, see notes. | 5-10 breaths | Thread the Needle - Lower Body page 127 |
| Seated Splits page 122 | Sit with your legs apart as wide as you can comfortably go, with toes pointing up. Lean forward and grab your toes or place your forearms on the floor. | 5-10 breaths | |
| Happy Baby page 123 | Lie on your back and grab the outside edges of your feet and rock side to side. | 5-10 breaths | |
| Pigeon page 130 | Bend your left leg so your shin is perpendicular to your body. Extend the back leg, keeping the hips level. Place your head on a block to relax, see notes. | 5-10 breaths and switch sides | |

# PRENATAL YOGA SEQUENCE - HIP OPENER CONTINUED

This sequence is excellent for opening the hips and releasing emotions and can be done right before bed and right when you wake up.

| Pose | Description | Breaths | Notes |
|---|---|---|---|
| Spinal Rotation page 128 | Lie on your back and bend your knees, with feet wide. Rotate the knees to one side. Place a block between the knees as shown in notes to reduce stress on the back. | 5-10 breaths and switch sides | |
| Figure 4 page 128 | From the position above, place the bottom heel on the top thigh. | 5-10 breaths and switch sides | |

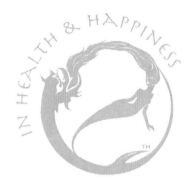

IN HEALTH & HAPPINESS

# PRENATAL YOGA SEQUENCE - UPPER BODY

# PRENATAL YOGA SEQUENCE - UPPER BODY

This sequence is excellent for strengthening and stretching the upper body as well as the back of the thighs and low back.

| Pose | Description | Breaths | Notes |
|---|---|---|---|
| Downward Dog page 133 | Press back into downward dog, trying to get your heels to the floor. If your heels do not go to the floor, bend your knees. Gaze toward your belly button. | Exhale and hold for 5 breaths, with long inhales and exhales | |
| Cat Pose page 118 | Come to all fours and round the back like a cat, as you exhale. | 1-5 breaths | |
| Cow Pose page 118 | Inhale and release the back like a cow. If this places stress on the low back come to table top pose shown in the notes section. | 1-5 breaths | Table Top page 118 |
| Thread the Needle - Upper Body page 127 | Place the left arm under the right and place the right hand on the floor, near your face. Press into the right palm twisting your body open to the right. Switch sides. | 5-10 breaths | |
| Child's Pose page 132 | Fold forward with feet together and knees wide to allow a place for your belly to drop. Extend your hands over head or place them by your sides. | 10 breaths, inhaling up the spine for 6 counts, hold for 2 counts at the top and exhaling down the spine for 6 counts. | |

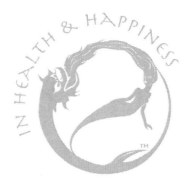

IN HEALTH & HAPPINESS

# SUN
# SALUTATION A

# PRENATAL SEQUENCE - SUN SALUTATION A

This sequence is excellent to helps revive you, pump fluid into your muscles and joints as well as warm you up for more strenuous poses.

| Pose | Description | Breaths | Notes |
|---|---|---|---|
| Mountain Pose page 136 | Stand with feet shoulder width apart and reach up to the sky, with palms together. | One breath - inhale | Lift the knee caps and squeeze the buttocks as you lightly draw the belly button in. |
| Standing Forward Bend page 137 | Swan dive forward and touch the floor with your palms or place your palms anywhere along your thighs that is comfortable. | One breath - exhale | |
| Half Standing Forward Bend page 138 | Look forward and come as close to a flat back as possible. | One breath - inhale | |
| Plank page 134 | Step your feet back to plank, on your toes or come to table to below. | One breath - exhale | |
| Table Top page 118 | Let yourself down into table top, coming back to all fours. | Continue to exhale | |

## SUN SALUTATION A CONTINUED

| Pose | Description | Breaths | Notes |
|---|---|---|---|
| Cow Pose page 118 | Inhale and press up to a cow or maintain table top position, with a slight lift of the head as in the notes section. | One breath - inhale | Table Top page 118 |
| Downward Dog page 133 | Press back into downward dog, trying to get your heels to the floor. If your heels do not go to the floor, bend your knees. Gaze toward your belly button. Come to child's pose if this is too strenuous, see notes. | Exhale and hold for 5 breaths, with long inhales and exhales | Childs Pose page 130 |
| Standing Forward Bend page 137 | Step or jump your feet forward, to a forward fold. | Inhale as you jump and exhale as you fold. | |
| Mountain Pose page 136 | Bending the knees come up slower than you want to, bringing your hands into prayer. | Inhale as you reach up and exhale as you bring the hands to prayer. | |

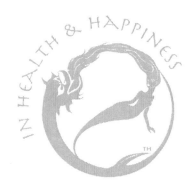

# LEG & BUTTOCKS STRENGTHENER SEQUENCE

# LEG AND BUTTOCKS STRENGTHENER SEQUENCE

It is ideal to warm up with 2-5 sun salutation A's prior to performing this sequence. This is an excellent sequence for keeping the legs and low back strong.

| Pose | Description | Breaths | Notes |
|------|-------------|---------|-------|
| Mountain Pose page 136 | Stand with hands in prayer feet together. | Hold for 1-5 breaths | |
| Warrior I page 144 | Step the left leg back and turn the toe out to 11:00 with the right foot at 12:00, Warrior I, knee tracking over second toe and in line with the ankle. Reach the arms up, legs and buttocks firm. If your left knee bothers you, lift the heel as shown in notes. | Exhale as you step back and inhale as you reach up. Hold for 1-5 breaths. | Crescent Lunge page 144 |
| Warrior II page 145 | Keeping the same stance, open the hips and turn the left foot to 9:00 and bend the right knee more deeply trying to get to a 90 degree angle, Warrior II. | Hold for 1-5 breaths | |

# LEG AND BUTTOCKS STRENGTHENER SEQUENCE CONTINUED

| Pose | Description | Breaths | Notes |
|---|---|---|---|
| Triangle Pose page 147 | With the right leg still forward, straighten the right leg and press the left hip back. Reach the right arm forward into triangle and lean back as if leaning against a wall. Raise the left arm up in line with right, jazz hand. | Hold for 1-5 breaths | |
| Downward Dog page 133 | Step back into Downward Dog. | Hold for 1-5 breaths | |
| Standing Forward Bend page 137 | Step or jump forward and fold in half. Inhale as you come forward and exhale as you fold. | Hold for 1-5 breaths | |
| Mountain Pose page 136 | Inhale, bend your knees slightly and slower than you want to, return to standing pose, hands in prayer or by your sides. Repeat sequence on the other side by stepping the right foot back. | Hold for 1-5 breaths | |

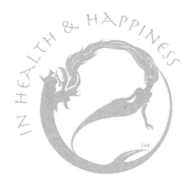

IN HEALTH & HAPPINESS

# NUTRITION

# 10 Tips For Prenatal Nutrition

- Why you should stay away from processed foods, nitrites and ingredients you cannot pronouce.
- Why you should avoid eating soy.
- Why you should avoid high fructose corn syrup.
- Why you should eat organic foods.
- What should you eat? Don't believe everything the media tells you.
- Why you should drink half you body weight in ounces of water a day.
- What foods are harmful to the baby.
- How to eat a healthy vegetarian diet.
- Which supplements you should take.
- Information on the effects of alcohol and caffeine on your baby.

## RESOURCES

1. www.westonaprice.org

2. www.savvyvegetarian.com

3. www.pregnancy.org

4. www.babycenter.com

5. *The Metabolic Typing Diet* by Dr. Wolcott and Trish Fahey

6. *How to Eat Move and Be Healthy!* by Paul Chek

7. Coryn Leaman, HHP - www.aohstore.com

8. *The Whole Soy Story* by Dr. Kaayla Daniels

9. *Nourishing Traditions* by Sally Fallon

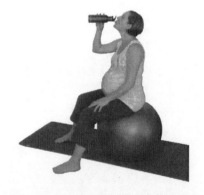

# Nutrition

## INTRODUCTION

This chapter will address how to eat healthy, giving your body the nutrients you need for a healthy pregnancy, allowing your baby to thrive. Many books recommend the food guide pyramid (now "Choose My Plate"[23]) as a nutritional guideline during pregnancy, with little guidance on anything else besides supplements. There is so much more to know about what we eat during pregnancy and the cause and effect of food on our bodies and our babies. Further, once your baby is born, it is important to feed your baby by making intelligent food choices based on the information discussed in *Postpartum Health and Happiness*.

First, I will explore the importance of avoiding processed foods and why organic foods are a better choice than commercial foods. Next we will look at "Choose My Plate" [23](formally the food guide pyramid) and why you should consider a nutritional plan that is not based solely on these resources. So much misinformation is out there regarding nutrition, which often times is driven by unreliable research studies, conducted by the very people trying to sell you something.

My goal is to help you make wise food choices, based on unbiased research, but not easily found in mainstream publications, because it does not generate revenue.

**Note:** A majority of the information sited in this chapter is found in research done by the Weston A. Price Foundation[20], Sally Fallon and Mary G. Enig, PhD[9]., Paul Chek, HHP[6] and Dr. William Wolcott and Trish Fahey the authors of *The Metabolic Typing Diet*[25]. These pioneers in the health and nutrition industry have been instrumental in dispelling so many myths about the foods we eat.

# Processed Foods

Processed foods are full of chemicals, many of which are hidden under "artificial" or "natural flavors". The FDA does not require food additives, "generally regarded as safe" (GRAS), to be listed on a food label. All you see is "artificial flavor" or "natural flavoring" or "artificial color."

If you look at any item found in a box, that is flavored, such as salad dressing, canned or even frozen meals, you will see ingredients you cannot pronounce and the words "artificial flavoring," "natural flavoring" or "artificial coloring." That is a red flag telling you this food is loaded with preservatives and chemicals that are harmful to you and your baby. Paul Chek[6] took a look at strawberry milkshake ingredients found at a fast food restaurant, ingredients not listed because they are GRAS and this is what he found:

> *Amyl acetate, amyl butyrate (additive in cigarettes), amyl valerate, anethol, anisyl formate, benzyl acetate, benzyl isobutyrate (found in fragrance and soap), butyric acid, cinnamyl isobutyrate, cinnamyl valerate, cognac essential oil, diacetyl, dipropyl, ketone, ethyl butyrate, ethyl cinnamate, ethyl heptanoate, ethyl lactate, ethyl methylphenlglycidate, ethyl nitrate, ethyl propionate, ethyl valerate, heliotropin, hydroxphrenyl-2 butanone (10% solution in alcohol), insert square–ionone, isobutyl anthranilate, isobutyl butrate, lemon essential oil, maltol, 4-nethylacetphenone, methyl anthranilate, methyl benzoate, methyl cinnamate, methyl heptine carbonate, methyl naphthyl ketone, methyl salicylate, mint essential oil, neroli essential oil, nerolin, neryl isobutyrate, orris butter, phenethyl alcohol, rose, rum ether, insert square-undecalactone, vanillin and solvent!.*

The reason I included this here is to send a message to you that processed foods are far more toxic than you can imagine. Simply plug anyone of those names you cannot pronounce into Google and see what you find out about its use. For example; According to Wikipedia, Ethyl butyrate, also known as ethyl butanoate, or butyric ether, is an ester with the chemical formula $CH_3CH_2CH_2COOCH_2CH_3$. It is soluble in propylene glycol, paraffin oil, and kerosene. It has a fruity odor, similar to pineapple[24].

Research conducted by Weston A. Price and Francis Marrion Pottenger[20] has linked disease with the consumption of processed foods. For more information I highly recommend you read "Pottenger's Cats" or "Nutrition and Physical Degeneration."

**Other things to consider when looking at processed foods are the following:**

## NITRITE

Nitrite is commonly found in packaged meats and fish. According to "The Safe Shopper's Bible", researchers reported that children who ate hot dogs cured with nitrite a dozen or more times monthly, have a risk of leukemia ten times higher than normal. Furthermore, children born to mothers who consume hotdogs once or more weekly during their pregnancy are twice as likely to have childhood brain tumors[6].

## SOY

Soy milk and soy products consumed in large quantities can cause the body a great deal of harm. According to the Weston A. Price Foundation[20], soy has the following dangers and side effects associated with it; reduces the absorption of key minerals in the diet, such as calcium, magnesium, iron and zinc, as well as increases the body's need for vitamin D. Most soy products contain MSG and aluminum, which are highly toxic to the nervous system. Not only is it a poor food choice for you, it is a poor food choice when deciding what to feed your baby. See the vegetarian section on page 209 and the postpartum section on formula and soy in *Postpartum Health and Happiness*.

# HIGH FRUCTOSE CORN SYRUP

Do not let anyone tell you that high fructose corn syrup is getting an undeserved bad rap. Manufactures use High Fructose Corn Syrup (HFCS) because it is extremely soluble and mixes well in many foods. It is cheap to produce, very sweet, and easy to store. It's used in everything from bread to pasta sauces to bacon to beer. It's even used in "health products" like protein/energy bars and "natural" sodas, so beware.[20]

High fructose corn syrup is often derived from genetically modified corn "involving vats of murky fermenting liquid, fungus and chemical tweaking"[10]. According to Dr. Mark Hyman[11], high fructose corn syrup is not a sugar the body recognizes and often bypasses the digestion process since there is no chemical bond between them. Therefore, they are more rapidly absorbed into your blood stream. Fructose goes right to the liver and triggers lipogenesis (the production of fats like triglycerides and cholesterol). This is why it is the major cause of liver damage in this country and causes a condition called "fatty liver", which affects 70 million people. The rapidly absorbed glucose triggers big spikes in insulin – our body's major fat storage hormone. Both these features of HFCS lead to increased metabolic disturbances that drive increases in appetite, weight gain, diabetes, heart disease, cancer and much more. For more information see the complete article at http://drhyman.com/blog/conditions/5-reasons-high-fructose-corn-syrup-will-kill-you/[11].

**Why are the side effects of high fructose corn syrup so devastating?** According to research done by the Weston A. Price foundation[20], not only does fructose have more damaging effects in the presence of copper deficiency, but fructose also inhibits copper metabolism--another example of the sweeteners double-whammy effect. A deficiency in copper leads to bone fragility, anemia, defects of the connective tissue, arteries, and bone, infertility, heart arrhythmias, high cholesterol levels, heart attacks, and an inability to control blood sugar levels. This is only one side effect of high fructose corn syrup. **To avoid high fructose corn syrup, choose foods that have natural cane sugar or organic sugar.**

# ARTIFICIAL SWEETENERS

The FDA has approved 5 non-nutritive sweeteners: aspartame, saccharin, acesulfame K, sucralose and neotame.[9] The most widely used non-nutritive sweetener is aspartame.

Problems associated with aspartame consumption are neatly summarized in Nourishing Traditions[9]. "Aspartame. . . is a neurotoxic substance that has been associated with numerous health problems including dizziness, visual impairment, severe muscle aches, numbing of extremities, pancreatitis, high blood pressure, retinal hemorrhaging, seizures and depression. It is suspected of causing birth defects and chemical disruptions in the brain.[9] If you want to avoid sugar, try using Stevia instead of artificial sweeteners.

# CARRAGEENAN

Carrageenan is a gel derived from red seaweeds. It coats the insides of the stomach, like gooey honey or massage oil. It is found in most lunch meats, cheeses, creams, milk to name a few products. Even the organic lunch meats, cheeses, milks and creams use carrageenan to give it creamier texture and taste. It has been found that digestive problems often occur from ingesting carrageenan. According to notmilk.com[7], Dr. Tobacman (a professor at the University of Iowa College of Medicine) shared studies with editor Robert Cohen that demonstrated that digestive enzymes and bacterial action, convert high weight carrageenans to dangerous low molecular weight carrageenans and poligeenans in the human gut. These carrageenans have been linked to various human cancers and digestive disorders. It is important to note that Tobacman's evidence and conclusions are based upon human tissue samples, not animal studies.[7]

Hopefully you are starting to see how so many ingredients that we think of as safe, can be harmful. Of course, in reality, it is not always easy to avoid processed foods. Especially when you have those pregnancy cravings. A simple rule of thumb to follow is, to eat well 80% of the time and your body can absorb the other 20%.[6] Read labels, if you eat processed foods, make sure they are organic, have ingredients you can pronounce and are not loaded with artificial and natural flavors or food coloring. Shop the perimeter of the store, where foods are fresh and wholesome. Avoid microwaves and use stainless steel cookware. Page 187 has a table on how to make healthier choices when you are having "junk" food cravings.

# ORGANIC VERSUS COMMERCIAL

There is so much hype out there now about organic foods. Are they really better? The answer is yes! Commercial foods are riddled with chemicals, "natural flavoring", growth hormones, antibiotics etc. The closer you are to finding foods that cavemen ate, the better off you and your baby will be. There are several reasons to eat organic: they are higher in nutrients, have little or no pesticides, chemical fertilizers or herbicides and they support a healthier environment.

## Higher Nutrient Value

The nutritional value is higher in organic foods. Most studies the media parades in front of us simply look at "primary nutrients" such as fats, water, fiber, protein, carbohydrates, vitamins and minerals. Yet the secondary nutrients are left out of many studies, which are what organic foods have much more of than commercial foods. Secondary nutrients contain phenolic compounds, which are a group of antioxidants that have been known to "mop up cancer-causing free radicals in the body"[6]. Further, numerous studies have found that organic foods contain far more vitamins, minerals, trace minerals, protein and enzymes than commercial foods.

## Organic Foods Have Fewer Toxins

Not only do organic foods have fewer toxins, they have less of an impact on the environment. According to the research cited in articles by Paul Chek[6], conventionally grown foods are laden with chemicals and pesticides such as chlorpyrifos, captan, iprodione and vinclozolin. These chemicals are carcinogenic and some have been linked to genetic and immune system damage. According to Goldsmith, one of the greatest ecologists of our time, "Literature linking cancer to exposure to carcinogenic chemicals is voluminous. According to WHO, solvents used in paints are known carcinogens, painters have a 40 percent higher chance of contracting stomach, bladder, larynx and other cancers, while their children are at increased risk of contracting leukemia and brain tumors." (www.edwardgoldsmith.org)[6]. These carcinogenic chemicals are put on the foods you and your baby are eating. Do your research. Plug any of these chemicals into google and see what you find.

Organic foods are better for the environment, as tons upon tons of pesticides and chemicals are not polluting the soil. Your food source is only as good as the soil it comes from.

A huge complaint about organic foods is the high price, yet in some markets, organic foods cost the same or pennies more. Many local growers sell pesticide free foods that may not be labeled organic, but are close in nutritional values and cost less. Remember, organic foods are so nutrient dense you need to eat less of them to satisfy your nutritional needs. Eating organic is preventative medicine. So when choosing foods from the "What to Eat" section, always choose organic whenever possible, and... Remember the 80/20 rule, if you eat well 80% of the time, your body can absorb 20% of the undesirable and harmful foods you eat[6].

# GENERAL FOODS MOST BOOKS TELL YOU TO AVOID

These foods have been known to be contaminated with listeria and should be avoided. See *What to Expect When You're Expecting*[16] for a more detailed list.
- Soft cheeses (brie, blue cheeses, Mexican style cheeses)
- Pate, cold cuts (salami, bologna, corned beef, liverwurst)

Other Foods To Avoid Due To Bacteria or Parasites
- Raw meats or fish (always cook thoroughly, even eggs)
- Alfalfa sprouts

# WHAT TO EAT?

Now that we have a good idea of what you should avoid, what should you eat? Growing a baby inside you takes a great deal of energy, calories and the right nutrients. This chapter identifies what foods are ideal to help you and your baby grow strong and healthy.

The first part of the nutrition section looks at the "Choose My Plate"[23](previously the food guide pyramid) as a source recommended by most books and articles out there for pregnant women to follow during their pregnancy and why this may not be the right diet for you to follow. Unconventional nutritional views will be explored and detailed information will be given to you to help you make the best dietary choices for you and your baby. As your body changes during pregnancy, you will crave foods you never wanted in the past and avoid foods you love. Some of the food cravings are unhealthy, so it is important to listen to your pregnancy cravings and try to stay away from those foods not offering healthy nutrients for you or your baby and seek a healthier alternative. A good rule of thumb is to, "step away from the sweets," and give yourself a few minutes to discover what your body is actually trying to tell you.

Here are some tips on listening to what your body is asking for and making healthier choices:

| Craving | Healthy Alternative |
|---------|---------------------|
| Sweet chocolate or cookies | Banana-chocolate smoothie with organic milk and coconut oil |
| Fast food hamburger - *most contain "pink slime" | Grilled burger or grilled chicken thigh or breast or nitrite free organic lunch meat and corn cakes |
| Tart candy like sour gummies | Spinach salad with green apples and cranberries |
| Salty foods like potato chips | Bake potatoes or sweet potato with sea salt or make your own fried potatoes in coconut oil or organic air popped popcorn with grass-fed butter like Kerrygold |
| Ice cream | Organic milk or ice cream smoothie with berries |
| Candy | Sweet fruits like berries, pineapples or peaches |
| Donuts or pastry | Sprouted toast with organic butter and jam |
| Sugar coated cereal | Organic oatmeal with brown sugar or pure maple syrup |

Table 1: Craving alternatives

*According to today's New York Times, The "majority of hamburgers" now sold in the U.S. now contains fatty slaughterhouse trimmings "the industry once relegated to pet food and cooking oil," "typically including most of the material from the outer surfaces of the carcass" that contains "larger microbiological populations." This "nasty pink slime," as one FDA microbiologist called it, is now wrung in a centrifuge to remove the fat, and then treated with AMMONIA to "retard spoilage," and turned into "a mashlike substance frozen into blocks or chips."[19]

# Choose My Plate or Not?

### Are the "Choose My Plate" recommendations right for you?

The USDA recommends the "Choose My Plate"[23] as a resource for pregnant woman, with enhancement of prenatal supplements. On the web site they do give proportion suggestions dependent on your age, sex, and level of physical activity, www.choosemyplate.gov. These recommendations are very generic and do not mention food intolerances, organic foods or food additives.

Let's take a look at each recommendation and explore other options based on current research for each macronutrient.

## GRAINS

**First, let's take a look The USDA recommendations for grains:**
The USDA recommends any food made from wheat, rice, oats, cornmeal, barley or another cereal grain is considered a grain product. Bread, pasta, oatmeal, breakfast cereals, tortillas, and grits are examples of grain products. Grains are divided into 2 subgroups, Whole Grains and Refined Grains.

**Whole grains contain the entire grain kernel, the bran, germ, and endosperm.**
Examples include:
whole-wheat flour, bulgur (cracked wheat), oatmeal, whole cornmeal and brown rice

**Refined grains have been milled, a process that removes the bran and germ. This is done to give grains a finer texture and improve their shelf life, but it also removes dietary fiber, iron, and many B vitamins.**
Some examples of refined grain products are:
white flour, de-germed cornmeal, white bread, and white rice

Most refined grains are enriched.* This means certain B vitamins (thiamin, riboflavin, niacin, folic acid) and iron are added back after processing. Fiber is not added back to enriched grains. Check the ingredient list on refined grain products to make sure that the word "enriched" is included in the grain name. Some food products are made from mixtures of whole grains and refined grains.

* Note: Vitamins added "back into" foods are often difficult for the body to absorb and therefore have no nutritional value.

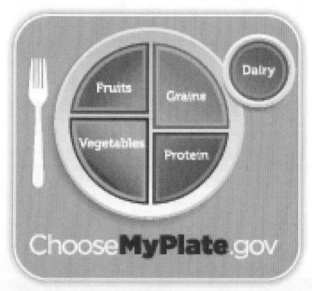

Illustration 8: ChooseMyPlate.gov

## What "ChooseMyPlate" does not tell you about grains:

Notice that most of the choices listed above for grains all contain wheat (gluten) except for brown rice. 50% of the population is intolerant to gluten. (Gluten (from Latin, gluten, "glue") is a protein composite found in foods processed from wheat and related grain species, including barley and rye). If you feel gassy and bloated after eating, experience constipation or runny stools and feel sluggish after eating foods containing gluten, you may be gluten intolerant. Remember that your body changes so much with pregnancy and what you could tolerate before pregnancy, you may no longer be able to tolerate and visa versa.

If you feel you may be gluten intolerant, you need to eliminate the following intolerable grains and replace them with tolerable grains.

| Intolerable Foods (contain gluten and gliadin) | Tolerable Foods |
| --- | --- |
| Wheat | Corn (non GMO) |
| Oats | Rice (rice pasta) and wild rice* |
| Couscous | Buckwheat |
| Quinoa | Millet |
| Barley | Arrowroot |
| Rye | Tapioca |
| Teff | Taro |
| Kamut | Wheat grass |
| Spelt | Barley grass |
| Amaranth | Barley malt |

Table 2: Gluten intolerable and tolerable foods

**Note:** Fermented soy products (e.g. tempe, tofu) contain high concentrations of soy protein, (which has 8 times the concentration of gliadin), which might make them problematic. See page 210 for more information on why you should avoid soy.

When eating any grains, it is best to avoid processed grains and eat sprouted grains when available. Further, not everyone needs to eat more grains than protein. Some people need to eat more protein than grains and in fact do better with very little grains. Keep a daily log of how you feel based on what you ate for at least a week. This will help you pin point foods that do not agree with you. For more information, refer to *The Metabolic Typing Diet* book by Dr. Wolcott[25].

*Consumer Reports showed high levels of arsenic were found in rice and should be avoided by pregnant women and infants. The guidelines stated to limit your intake to one serving of rice (or other rice products) per week for children and pregnant women and two servings for other adults. A serving is based on one-fourth cup of uncooked rice (which is about half a cup of cooked brown rice and about three-fourths cup to one cup cooked basmati).

# FRUITS AND VEGETABLES

According to "Choose My Plate", any vegetable or 100% vegetable juice counts as a member of the Vegetable Group. Vegetables may be raw or cooked; fresh, frozen, canned, or dried/dehydrated; and may be whole, cut-up, or mashed.

Vegetables are organized into 5 subgroups, based on their nutrient content.

- Dark green vegetables
- Starchy vegetables
- Red & orange vegetables
- Beans and peas
- Other vegetables

According to "ChooseMyPlate," any fruit or 100% fruit juice counts as part of the Fruit Group. Fruits may be fresh, canned, frozen, or dried, and may be whole, cut-up, or pureed.

## What "ChooseMyPlate" does not tell you about fruits and vegetables:

All fruits and vegetables are not created equally. Fruit and vegetable juices and canned fruits and vegetables are not a viable option. Most fruit and vegetable juices, as well as canned fruits and vegetables, often contain too much sodium and high fructose corn syrup and are dead; meaning they have no life in them.

Further, According to Natural Resources Defense Council (NRCD)[17], most produce grown in the United States travels an average of 1,500 miles before it gets sold. Trucking, shipping and flying in food from around the country and the globe takes a toll on the environment and on public health. Take grapes, for example, every year, nearly 270 million pounds of grapes arrive in California, most of them shipped from Chile to the Port of Los Angeles. Their 5,900 mile journey in cargo ships and trucks releases 7,000 tons of global warming pollution each year, and enough air pollution to cause dozens of asthma attacks and hundreds of missed school days in California.

The way we eat has an enormous impact on the health of the planet. By choosing to eat lower on the food chain, and focusing on local and organic produce, we can curb global warming and air pollution, avoid toxic pesticides, support local farmers and enjoy fresh, tasty food.

The following website will tell you when certain fruits and vegetables are in-season and where a farmer's market is in your area: www.nrdc.org/health/foodmiles and www.westonaprice.org[20].

I have included a sample from the NRDC website on fruits and vegetables and when they are in-season in California.

## Early January

Apples, Asparagus, Avocados, Beets, Bok Choy, Broccoli, Cabbage, Carrots, Cauliflower, Celery, Fennel, Grapefruit, Halibut, Pacific, Kale, Lettuce, Mushrooms, Okra, Onions, Oranges, Pears, Pistachios, Potatoes, Radishes, Rutabaga, Scallions, Shrimp, Pink, Spinach, Squash, Strawberries, Turnips

## Late January

Apples, Asparagus, Avocados, Beets, Bok Choy, Broccoli, Cabbage, Carrots, Cauliflower, Celery, Fennel, Grapefruit, Halibut, Pacific, Kale, Lettuce, Mushrooms, Okra, Onions, Oranges, Pears, Pistachios, Potatoes, Radishes, Rutabaga, Scallions, Shrimp, Pink, Spinach, Squash, Strawberries, Turnips

## Early February

Apples, Asparagus, Avocados, Beets, Bok Choy, Broccoli, Brussels Sprouts, Cabbage, Carrots, Cauliflower, Celery, Fennel, Grapefruit, Halibut, Pacific, Kale, Lettuce, Mushrooms, Okra, Onions, Oranges, Pears, Pistachios, Potatoes, Radishes, Rutabaga, Scallions, Shrimp, Pink, Spinach, Squash, Strawberries, Turnips

## Late February

Apples, Asparagus, Avocados, Beets, Bok Choy, Broccoli, Brussels Sprouts, Cabbage, Carrots, Cauliflower, Celery, Fennel, Grapefruit, Halibut, Pacific, Kale, Lettuce, Mushrooms, Okra, Onions, Oranges, Pears, Pistachios, Potatoes, Radishes, Rutabaga, Scallions, Shrimp, Pink, Spinach, Squash, Strawberries, Turnips

## Early March

Apples, Asparagus, Avocados, Beets, Bok Choy, Broccoli, Cabbage, Carrots, Cauliflower, Celery, Fennel, Grapefruit, Halibut, Pacific, Kale, Lettuce, Mushrooms, Okra, Onions, Oranges, Pistachios, Potatoes, Radishes, Rutabaga, Scallions, Shrimp, Pink, Spinach, Strawberries, Tomatoes, Turnips

## Late March

Apples, Asparagus, Avocados, Beets, Bok Choy, Broccoli, Cabbage, Carrots, Cauliflower, Celery, Fennel, Grapefruit, Halibut, Pacific, Kale, Lettuce, Mushrooms, Okra, Onions, Oranges, Pistachios, Potatoes, Radishes, Rutabaga, Scallions, Shrimp, Pink, Spinach, Strawberries, Tomatoes, Turnips

## Early April

Apples, Asparagus, Avocados, Beets, Bok Choy, Broccoli, Brussels Sprouts, Cabbage, Carrots, Cauliflower, Celery, Cherries, Fennel, Grapefruit, Halibut, Pacific, Kale, Lettuce, Mushrooms, Nectarines, Okra, Onions, Oranges, Peas, Pistachios, Potatoes, Radishes, Raspberries, Rhubarb, Rutabaga, Scallions, Shrimp, Pink, Spinach, Strawberries, Tomatoes, Turnips

## Late April

Apples, Asparagus, Avocados, Beets, Bok Choy, Broccoli, Cabbage, Carrots, Cauliflower, Celery, Cherries, Fennel, Grapefruit, Halibut, Pacific, Kale, Lettuce, Mushrooms, Nectarines, Okra, Onions, Oranges, Peas, Pistachios, Potatoes, Radishes, Raspberries, Rhubarb, Rutabaga, Scallions, Shrimp, Pink, Spinach, Strawberries, Tomatoes, Turnips

## Early May

Apples, Apricots, Asian Pears, Asparagus, Avocados, Beets, Blackberries, Bok Choy, Broccoli, Cabbage, Carrots, Cauliflower, Celery, Cherries, Cucumbers, Eggplant, Fennel, Grapefruit, Halibut, Pacific, Kale, Lettuce, Mushrooms, Nectarines, Okra, Onions, Oranges, Peaches, Peas, Pistachios, Potatoes, Radishes, Raspberries, Rhubarb, Scallions, Spinach, Squash, Strawberries, Tomatoes

## Late May

Apples, Apricots, Asian Pears, Asparagus, Avocados, Beets, Blackberries, Blueberries, Bok Choy, Broccoli, Cabbage, Carrots, Cauliflower, Celery, Cherries, Cucumbers, Eggplant, Fennel, Grapefruit, Halibut, Pacific, Kale, Lettuce, Mushrooms, Nectarines, Okra, Onions, Oranges, Peaches, Peas, Pistachios, Potatoes, Radishes, Raspberries, Rhubarb, Scallions, Spinach, Squash, Strawberries, Tomatoes

## Early June

Apples, Apricots, Asian Pears, Asparagus, Avocados, Beets, Blackberries, Blueberries, Bok Choy, Broccoli, Cabbage, Carrots, Cauliflower, Celery, Cherries, Cucumbers, Eggplant, Fennel, Grapefruit, Halibut, Pacific, Kale, Lettuce, Mushrooms, Nectarines, Okra, Onions, Oranges, Peaches, Pears, Peas, Pistachios, Radishes, Raspberries, Rhubarb, Scallions, Snap Peas, Spinach, Squash, Strawberries, Tomatoes

## Late June

Apples, Apricots, Asian Pears, Asparagus, Avocados, Beets, Blackberries, Blueberries, Bok Choy, Broccoli, Cabbage, Carrots, Cauliflower, Celery, Cherries, Cucumbers, Eggplant, Fennel, Grapefruit, Grapes, Halibut, Pacific, Kale, Lettuce, Mushrooms, Nectarines, Okra, Onions, Oranges, Peaches, Pears, Peas, Pistachios, Radishes, Raspberries, Rhubarb, Scallions, Snap Peas, Spinach, Squash, Strawberries, Tomatoes

## Early July

Apples, Apricots, Asian Pears, Asparagus, Avocados, Beets, Blackberries, Blueberries, Broccoli, Cabbage, Carrots, Cauliflower, Celery, Cherries, Cucumbers, Eggplant, Fennel, Grapefruit, Grapes, Halibut, Pacific, Lettuce, Mushrooms, Nectarines, Okra, Onions, Oranges, Peaches, Pears, Peas, Pistachios, Potatoes, Radishes, Raspberries, Rhubarb, Scallions, Snap Peas, Spinach, Squash, Strawberries, Tomatoes

## Late July

Apples, Apricots, Asian Pears, Asparagus, Avocados, Beets, Blackberries, Blueberries, Broccoli, Brussels Sprouts, Cabbage, Carrots, Celery, Cherries, Cucumbers, Eggplant, Fennel, Grapefruit, Grapes, Halibut, Pacific, Lettuce, Mushrooms, Nectarines, Okra, Onions, Oranges, Peaches, Pears, Peas, Pistachios, Potatoes, Radishes, Raspberries, Rhubarb, Scallions, Snap Peas, Spinach, Squash, Strawberries, Tomatoes

## Early August

Apples, Asian Pears, Asparagus, Avocados, Beets, Broccoli, Brussels Sprouts, Cabbage, Carrots, Celery, Cucumbers, Eggplant, Fennel, Grapefruit, Grapes, Halibut, Pacific, Lettuce, Mushrooms, Nectarines, Okra, Onions, Oranges, Peaches, Pears, Peas, Pistachios, Potatoes, Radishes, Raspberries, Rhubarb, Scallions, Snap Peas, Spinach, Squash, Strawberries, Tomatoes

## Late August

Apples, Asian Pears, Asparagus, Avocados, Beets, Broccoli, Brussels Sprouts, Cabbage, Carrots, Celery, Cucumbers, Eggplant, Fennel, Grapefruit, Grapes, Halibut, Pacific, Lettuce, Mushrooms, Nectarines, Okra, Onions, Oranges, Peaches, Pears, Peas, Pistachios, Potatoes, Radishes, Raspberries, Rhubarb, Scallions, Snap Peas, Spinach, Squash, Strawberries, Tomatoes

## Early September

Apples, Asian Pears, Asparagus, Avocados, Beets, Bok Choy, Broccoli, Brussels Sprouts, Cabbage, Carrots, Cauliflower, Celery, Cucumbers, Eggplant, Fennel, Grapefruit, Grapes, Halibut, Pacific, Kale, Lettuce, Mushrooms, Nectarines, Okra, Onions, Oranges, Peaches, Pears, Peas, Pistachios, Potatoes, Radishes, Raspberries, Rhubarb, Scallions, Snap Peas, Spinach, Squash, Strawberries, Sweet Potatoes, Tomatoes, Turkey - Bourbon Red, Turkey - Standard Bronze, Turnips

## Late September

Apples, Asian Pears, Asparagus, Avocados, Beets, Bok Choy, Broccoli, Brussels Sprouts, Cabbage, Carrots, Cauliflower, Celery, Cucumbers, Eggplant, Fennel, Grapefruit, Grapes, Halibut, Pacific, Kale, Lettuce, Mushrooms, Nectarines, Okra, Onions, Oranges, Peaches, Pears, Peas, Pistachios, Potatoes, Radishes, Raspberries, Rhubarb, Scallions, Snap Peas, Spinach, Squash, Strawberries, Sweet Potatoes, Tomatoes, Turkey - Bourbon Red, Turkey - Standard Bronze, Turnips

## Early October

Apples, Asian Pears, Asparagus, Avocados, Beets, Bok Choy, Broccoli, Brussels Sprouts, Cabbage, Carrots, Cauliflower, Celery, Cucumbers, Eggplant, Fennel, Grapefruit, Grapes, Halibut, Pacific, Kale, Lettuce, Mushrooms, Nectarines, Okra, Onions, Oranges, Peaches, Pears, Peas, Pistachios, Potatoes, Radishes, Raspberries, Rhubarb, Rutabaga, Scallions, Snap Peas, Spinach, Squash, Strawberries, Sweet Potatoes, Tomatoes, Turkey - Bourbon Red, Turkey - Standard Bronze, Turnips

## Late October

Apples, Asian Pears, Asparagus, Avocados, Beets, Bok Choy, Broccoli, Brussels Sprouts, Cabbage, Carrots, Cauliflower, Celery, Cucumbers, Eggplant, Fennel, Grapefruit, Grapes, Halibut, Pacific, Kale, Lettuce, Mushrooms, Nectarines, Okra, Onions, Oranges, Peaches, Pears, Peas, Pistachios, Potatoes, Radishes, Raspberries, Rhubarb, Rutabaga, Scallions, Snap Peas, Spinach, Squash, Strawberries, Sweet Potatoes, Tomatoes, Turkey - Bourbon Red, Turkey - Standard Bronze, Turnips

## Early November

Apples, Asparagus, Avocados, Beets, Bok Choy, Broccoli, Brussels Sprouts, Cabbage, Carrots, Cauliflower, Celery, Cucumbers, Eggplant, Fennel, Grapefruit, Grapes, Halibut, Pacific, Kale, Lettuce, Mushrooms, Okra, Onions, Oranges, Peaches, Pears, Peas, Pistachios, Potatoes, Radishes, Raspberries, Rhubarb, Rutabaga, Scallions, Shrimp, Pink, Snap Peas, Spinach, Squash, Sweet Potatoes, Tomatoes, Turkey - Bourbon Red, Turkey - Standard Bronze, Turnips

## Late November

Apples, Asparagus, Avocados, Beets, Bok Choy, Broccoli, Brussels Sprouts, Cabbage, Carrots, Cauliflower, Celery, Christmas Trees, Cucumbers, Eggplant, Fennel, Grapefruit, Grapes, Halibut, Pacific, Kale, Lettuce, Mushrooms, Okra, Onions, Oranges, Peaches, Pears, Peas, Pistachios, Potatoes, Radishes, Raspberries, Rhubarb, Rutabaga, Scallions, Shrimp, Pink, Snap Peas, Spinach, Squash, Sweet Potatoes, Tomatoes, Turkey - Bourbon Red, Turkey - Standard Bronze, Turnips, Wreathes

## Early December

Apples, Avocados, Beets, Bok Choy, Broccoli, Brussels Sprouts, Cabbage, Carrots, Cauliflower, Celery, Christmas Trees, Cucumbers, Fennel, Grapefruit, Grapes, Halibut, Pacific, Kale, Lettuce, Mushrooms, Okra, Onions, Oranges, Pears, Pistachios, Potatoes, Radishes, Rutabaga, Scallions, Shrimp, Pink, Snap Peas, Spinach, Squash, Sweet Potatoes, Tomatoes, Turkey - Bourbon Red, Turkey - Standard Bronze, Turnips, Wreathes

## Late December

Apples, Avocados, Beets, Bok Choy, Broccoli, Brussels Sprouts, Cabbage, Carrots, Cauliflower, Celery, Christmas Trees, Cucumbers, Fennel, Grapefruit, Grapes, Halibut, Pacific, Kale, Lettuce, Mushrooms, Okra, Onions, Oranges, Pears, Pistachios, Potatoes, Radishes, Rutabaga, Scallions, Shrimp, Pink, Snap Peas, Spinach, Squash, Sweet Potatoes, Tomatoes, Turkey - Bourbon Red, Turkey - Standard Bronze, Turnips, Wreathes

Lastly, fruits and vegetables are an excellent source of vitamins, but be sure to eat fruits and vegetables that are organic, are in season and eat them in moderation. Frozen organic fruits and vegetables are sometimes a better option, as they hold up better in transit. Fruits, and some vegetables, still have lots of sugar, so be careful how much you eat, especially if you have pregnancy induced diabetes.

Eating fruit with fat and protein, such as cheese, will help keep your blood sugar levels even. If you develop digestive issues, *The Metabolic Typing Diet* book[25] has a great resource on food combing to alleviate digestive issues.

## DAIRY

Dairy can be a very valuable part of your diet if you are not allergic or intolerant to dairy. Weston A. Price highly recommends raw dairy, as it still contains the enzymes needed to break down dairy in the gut. If you can handle cow dairy, then by all means go for it, making sure it is organic or raw dairy. If not, consider drinking goat's milk and eating goat and sheep dairy products. Goat and sheep milk seem to be a great, tolerable alternative to cow dairy when you are dairy intolerant. Be careful consuming soy as a dairy alternative, as soy products are very harmful to the body (see section on soy page 210).

## MEAT

Red meat has gotten a lot of bad press over the years. Beef is believed to cause heart disease, cancer, and to harbor E. coli, to name a few of its crimes. Most people tend to avoid beef, believing it will raise their blood serum cholesterol and therefore increase their risk of heart disease. If you watch the trends of human consumption over the past eighty years, it is true that beef consumption has gone up, as well as heart disease. However, the media fails to show that though beef consumption has gone up 46% since 1909, poultry consumption has gone up 280%, vegetable oil consumption is up 437% and butter and lard consumption has decreased from 30 pounds per person per year to just under 10 pounds. Most of the foods believed to cause heart disease are being consumed less and those believed to have no correlation to consumption and heart diseases are consumed more. Sally Fallon states, "The most likely causes of increased heart disease in America are the other changes in our diet, huge increases in consumption of refined carbohydrates and vegetable oils, particularly hydrogenated vegetable oils; and the decline in nutrient levels in our food, particularly minerals and fat soluble vitamins-vitamins found only in animal fats."[20]

Of course, the source of any meat is important. Organic, grass-fed beef is the only way to insure that the quality of fat found in the meat contains the vitamins and minerals we need. Check with your local butcher to make sure the meat you are getting is chemical free, hormone free and all ground beef, chicken or turkey is ground fresh at the butcher shop. You don't want beef that contains "pink slime."[19]

Eggs should also be organic, hormone free and from free-range chickens. If you are allergic or intolerant to grains, try to find local eggs from chickens that are fed only vegetables and non-gmo corn. To know if an egg is good, the shell should be hard and if you place a raw egg in a large bowl of cold water, it should sink. Yolks should be a deep yellow or orange. You may have a local egg farm close by; we do and we live in a rural area, so be sure to check around.

# GELATIN

Gelatin has been shown to improve digestion and reduce inflammation. Gelatin is comprised of all the stuff we no longer use when eating an animal. We simply eat the meat and discard the bones, tendons and ligaments. According to Ray Peat "Gelatin (the cooked form of collagen) makes up about 50% of the protein in an animal, but a much smaller percentage in the more active tissues, such as brain, muscle, and liver. 35% of the amino acids in gelatin are glycine, 11% alanine, and 21% proline and hydroxyproline. In the industrialized societies, the consumption of gelatin has decreased, relative to the foods that contain an inappropriately high proportion of the antimetabolic amino acids, especially tryptophan and cysteine. The degenerative and inflammatory diseases can often be corrected by the use of gelatin-rich foods". For more information go to raypeat.com.

Consider adding 4-8 tablespoons of gelatin to your diet a day. A good source of gelatin is Great lakes.

Gelatin Facts from Great Lakes: Great Lakes Web Site - www.greatlakes.com

1.  Our Gelatin and Hydrolysate contains no MSG. Some believe that Glutamic acid or Mono sodium glutamate is contained in gelatin. This is simply not the case.

2.  Our products are all gluten free. Gelatin and related products from Great lakes Gelatin are totally free from gluten. Glutens are the proteins found in wheat, barley and rye flours (all Triticeae plants). Wheat glutens are a problem for a small group of individuals who have allergies to these proteins (primarily for persons suffering from celiac disease). Glutens are plant derived proteins. Gelatin is produced entirely from animals and contains absolutely no gluten.

3.  Gelatin is a natural occurring protein. The raw material used for production of gelatin is the naturally occurring protein collagen which is commercially sourced from the meat industry from healthy animals designated for human consumption. Each stage of the manufacturing process is rigorously controlled in modern laboratories to ensure purity and quality. The process of converting collagen into gelatine involves several cleansing and purification steps. The end result is an off white dry powder of the utmost purity.

## Orange Gelatin
Use organic ingredients whenever possible.
*   4 tablespoons great lakes gelatin (Great Lakes Gelatin)
*   4 cups orange juice (for variety, substitute one cup orange juice with one cup cranberry juice)
*   Gently boil 2 cups of juice

Stir 4 tablespoons of gelatin into 2 cups of cold juice, for 3 minutes, making sure it dissolves completely.
Slowly add boiling juice and stir until completely mixed.
Refrigerate for 4-6 hours until hard.
Makes an excellent snack full of much needed protein.

## Bone Broth:
Use chicken feet or beef knuckles for the best broth. It is important the bones you use have a lot of marrow.
1 quart water per pound of bones
1-2 Tablespoons Orange juice/Vinegar

Boil 5-6 hours and strain bones
Refrigerate and then remove layer of fat from top and discard
Drink 8-16 ounces a day.

## BEANS

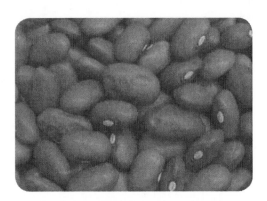

Researchers tested the antioxidant activity of flavonoids found in the skin of 12 varieties of dry beans. Antioxidants are known to destroy free radicals and help prevent heart disease, cancer and aging. Following the study, researchers found that black beans had the most antioxidants, followed by red, brown, yellow and white beans. The darker the bean is, the higher the level of flavonoids it contains, and therefore the higher antioxidant activity it has.

When buying beans in a can, read the sodium levels. Sodium levels in canned foods are high, plus, canned food is dead and should be avoided. The best way to get the most nutrients out of your beans is to buy them dry and soak them overnight before cooking. Simmer over low heat for 4 hours. Soaking beans help you digest them better and make a more "complete" protein. Adding salt is great, but make sure that it is sea salt or Himalayan salt, as it will contain all the minerals needed by the body. Never use table salt or iodized salt. The more color the salt, has the richer in nutrients it is, because it has not been bleached and striped of minerals.[6]

Should you choose not to eat meat, beans are a valuable source to make complete proteins in our bodies.

Below are some ideas of what to eat beans with to get the most protein in your diet.

- Black beans and rice
- Nuts and seeds plus legumes
- Lentil soup with a serving of almonds on the side
- Corn plus legumes. Try pinto beans in a corn tortilla.
- Try whole grain pasta or rice pasta, tossed with peas, almonds, and your favorite sauce.
- Whole wheat toast or Ezekiel sprouted toast with peanut butter will give you a complete protein.
- Bean soup with whole grain crackers.
- Corn tortillas with refried beans and rice.
- Grains plus legumes.

# Important Nutrients that do Not Appear on "Choose My Plate" that Should

## Fats

Your body needs fats, but the source needs to be a good one as discussed under the topic of meats and beans. Saturated fats have also been deemed "unhealthy" and "a cause of heart disease". Saturated fats from good meat sources are not only healthy, but they are vital for enhancing the immune system, are necessary for healthy bones, protect the liver, do not go rancid when heated to high heats, do not call upon the body's reserve of anti-oxidants, do not initiate cancer, and do not irritate artery walls.[20]

Consuming good fats is especially important when you are trying to get pregnant to insure that your body has the necessary building blocks to make the needed reproductive hormones. It continues to be important during pregnancy and breastfeeding, as your body continues to make hormones to nourish your baby.

Butter is better. Butter protects us against many diseases in the same way that red meat does. Butter is believed to cause heart disease, yet again, as the incidence of heart disease rose, the consumption of butter decreased. Butter contains many nutrients we need to protect us from heart disease such as Vitamin A (see page 205), as well as lecithin, which assists in the proper assimilation and metabolism of cholesterol and other fat constituents.

Further, Dr. Weston A. Price[20] discovered the X-factor, found in butter and animal fat, (now believed to be vitamin K2) that is also essential for optimal growth. It is a powerful catalyst which, like vitamins A and D, helps the body absorb and utilize minerals. According to the Weston A. Price foundation, "A growing body of published research confirms Dr. Price's discoveries, namely that vitamin K2 is important for the utilization of minerals, protects against tooth decay, supports growth and development, is involved in normal reproduction, protects against calcification of the arteries leading to heart disease, and is a major component of the brain. Butter is also essential for the development of children. It plays a vital role in brain development and nervous system development from inception to adulthood".[20]

Butter is also a good source of antioxidants and cholesterol. The bottom line is; do not throw your butter away in exchange for margarine containing highly processed rancid vegetable oils, soy protein and a bunch of other additives. Some margarine still contains hydrogenated fats.

If you have a hard time eating butter or getting your child to eat butter, add the X-Factor Gold™ High-Vitamin Butter Oil found at www.building-health.com to a smoothie. Butter is a great resource for those who cannot stomach organ meats that are high in vitamin A.

# Other Important Types of Fat

The following information on important fats we need in our diets and where to get them is an exert from Paul Chek's book "How to Eat Move and Be Healthy."[6] This information is based on Paul Chek's thorough research. For more information "How To Eat, Move and Be Healthy"[6] can be found at www.chekinstitute.com.

## Saturated Fats

- Found in animal fats and tropical oils (organic palm and coconut are easiest to find)
- Do not normally go rancid even when heated for cooking
- Made in our bodies from carbohydrates
- Constitutes at least 50% of the cell membranes; they give cells stiffness and integrity
- Needed for calcium to effectively be incorporated into skeletal system
- Protect liver from alcohol and other toxins
- Enhance immune system
- Needed for proper use of EFAs (Essential Fatty Acids)

Sources: animal products, coconut and palm oil

## Monounsaturated Fats

- Tend to be liquid at room temperature
- Do not go rancid easily and can be used in cooking at moderate temperatures

Sources: olive oil, almonds, pecans, cashews, peanuts and avocados

## Polyunsaturated Fats

- Contain linoleic acid (omega 6) and linolenic acid (omega 3) - essential because our bodies cannot produce them
- Liquid, even when refrigerated
- Should never be heated

Sources: vegetable oils, fish oil, eggs and walnuts

## FATS TO AVOID

Trans-fatty acids (TFA) and hydrogenated or partially hydrogenated oils should be avoided, as they are hard for the body to assimilate and use. Structurally, trans-fatty acids are closer to plastic than fat. TFA consumption has been linked to heart disease and elevated cholesterol levels. TFAs are also thought to impair lipoprotein receptors in cells, impairing the body's ability to process low-density cholesterol (LDL), increasing their rate of synthesis and eventually elevating LDL levels in the blood. (LDL's are considered the "bad" cholesterol as it has a tendency to build up in the inner walls of the arteries, causing a narrowing of the arterial walls (atherosclerosis).

## Samples of Foods containing trans-fatty acids are:

- Margarine
- Any product with ingredients that say "not a significant source of trans-fatty acids" - a very interesting article can be found on http://www.bantransfats.com/faq.html regarding the "oreo cookie case" back in 2003.[20]

# Cholesterol

Before you believe everything you hear about cholesterol, do your research. My doctor tried to put me on a cholesterol lowering medication while I was breastfeeding because my cholesterol was too high. Of course it was high, it needed to be. If I had not taken the time to research the false information out there about cholesterol levels, I may have taken a statin drug while breastfeeding, which would not only harm me, but reduce the amount of much needed cholesterol in my milk and pass on dangerous chemicals to my baby. DO YOUR RESEARCH. The following information is taken directly from an article by Sally Fallon at www.westonaprice.org/mythstruths/mtbeef.html. I decided to place the entire 2 paragraphs in this manual, as nobody says it better than Sally Fallon[9].

"The truth is that cholesterol is your best friend. It is vital for the function of the nervous system and the integrity of the digestive tract. Steroid hormones that help the body deal with stress are made from cholesterol. Sex hormones like estrogen and testosterone are made from cholesterol. Bile salts that the body uses to digest fats are made from cholesterol. Vitamin D, needed for thousands of biochemical processes, is made from cholesterol.

Cholesterol is a powerful antioxidant that protects us against cancer. It is vital to the cells because it provides waterproofing and structural integrity. And, finally, cholesterol is the body's repair substance. When our arteries are weak and develop fissures or tears, cholesterol is sequestered and used for repair. When cholesterol levels in the blood are high, it's because the body needs cholesterol. Blaming heart disease on cholesterol is like blaming a fire on the fireman who arrives to put out the flames."[9]

Remember that low levels of cholesterol can be much more dangerous than high levels. According to Sally Fallon, "people with cholesterol levels lower than 180 are at a greater risk of death from other causes, such as cancer, intestinal disease, accidents, violence and suicide." [9]

If blood serum cholesterol is high, it is better to find out why instead of putting a band-aid on it with statin drugs. The side effects of statins are extremely dangerous and life altering and most times physicians are giving them to patients for "prevention." An article in the Union Tribune cited numerous doctors who are given kickbacks and vacations that are fully paid for by pharmaceutical companies in exchange for pushing their cholesterol lowering drugs. We live in a time where we need to question what our doctors tell us, as the motive behind their diagnosis may not always be honest.

## Benefits of Cholesterol

- Gives cells stiffness and stability
- Is a precursor to steroid hormones and vitamin D
- Is needed for proper function of serotonin receptors in brain
- Acts as an antioxidant
- Low cholesterol levels have been linked to aggressive and violent behavior, depression and suicidal tendencies
- Has a role in maintaining the health of the intestinal wall
- High-serum cholesterol levels often indicate that the body needs cholesterol to protect itself from high levels of altered free-radical-containing fats

Sources: animal products

## OMEGA-3 FATTY ACIDS

The following information is in part resourced from the American Journal of Clinical Nutrition, Vol. 71, No. 1, 171S-175S, January 2000 (http://www.ajcn.org/content/71/1/171S.abstract).[3]

During pregnancy, both maternal stores and dietary intake of omega-3 fatty acids are of importance in insuring that the baby has adequate amounts of omega-3 fatty acids at the time of birth. All the polyunsaturated fatty acids, including DHA, are transferred across the placenta into fetal blood. In addition, EPA and DHA in maternal adipose tissue (fat cells) can be made available to the developing fetus via placenta transport.

### DHA

Docosahexaenoic acid (DHA) is an omega-3 fatty acid that is a primary structural component of the human brain cerebral cortex, sperm, testicles and retina.[24]

### EPA

Eicosapentaenoic acid (EPA or also icosapentaenoic acid) is an omega-3 fatty acid. It is obtained in the human diet by eating oily fish or fish oil - e.g., cod liver, herring, mackerel, salmon, menhaden and sardine. It is also found in human breast milk.[24]

However, fish do not naturally produce EPA, but obtain it from the algae they consume.

Several studies in monkeys have indicated that when the maternal diet is deficient in omega-3 fatty acids, the infant at birth is likewise deficient, as evidenced by low DHA concentrations in their plasma and red blood cells.

In humans, it was shown that the administration of fish oil or sardines to pregnant women led to higher DHA concentrations in both maternal plasma and red blood cells and in cord blood plasma and red blood cells at the time of birth. Once membrane phospholipids have adequate concentrations of DHA, there is an avid retention of these fatty acids in the brain and the retina, even though the diet may subsequently be deficient. Several studies illustrate clearly the effects of omega-3 deficiency in both animals and humans. Further, studies have shown that higher levels of cod liver oil in the diet promote strong bones, immunity, normal growth, successful reproduction, good nervous system function, insulin production, healthy skin and good eyesight to list a few.[15] See page 206 for good sources of fish oil.

## COOKING OIL

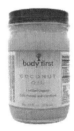

It is important to choose stable fats when cooking at high heats, such as coconut oil, ghee, palm oil and lard. For medium heat, you can use sesame oil, hazelnut oil and for low heat olive oil.

Oils that are good to take with no heat include olive oil and flax seed oil, (The flaxseed needs to be ground in order for the proper digestion of the seeds to take place.) Two tablespoons of flaxseed is about 20 grams of seed and since there is about 40 percent oil in the seeds and about 50-60 percent omega-3 in the oil, 20 grams of seed could provide about 8 grams of flaxseed oil and about 4 grams alpha-linolenic acid, the basic omega-3 fatty acid.

# Foods to Avoid

There are many resources telling pregnant women what to avoid. After reading several books, the general list of foods to avoid are mentioned below. It is best to avoid these foods because of the possibility of them containing listeriosis, a form of food poisoning or parasites:[10,16] Although we may be able to ward off parasites, a growing baby may not.

- Soft cheeses (feta, brie etc.)
- Pate
- Raw fish (can carry parasites that the fetus cannot fight off and places that serve raw fish may use the same knives to cut cooked food, so be careful when eating in these establishments).
- Raw shellfish (make sure all shellfish is fully cooked)
- Deli meats
- Hot dogs
- Under cooked poultry, red meat

# Water

Our bodies are 70-75% water. Water is essential for maintaining a stable environment inside and around our cells, allowing us to acquire sufficient nutrition and aiding in elimination of waste in cells. The placenta and amniotic fluid are dependent on how hydrated you are. Drinking half your body weight in ounces of water a day is important for the average person. When you are pregnant you should drink about 60% of your body weight in ounces of water a day to be on the safe side . So if you weigh 120 pounds, you need to drink 60-70 ounces of water a day. And as your weight increases, so do the ounces you consume.

## Source:

Make sure you are drinking water that is stored in a container that does not leak all sorts of plastic chemicals into the water. The water you are drinking should have a hardness factor of 170/mg/L or greater and a Total Dissolved Solids (TDS) of 300 or greater. Consider buying a water filtration system for the house or use a filter system sold in most camping stores to filter your water.

One of the best ways to carry your water around with you, and for your future child, is using a steel container such as Klean Kanteen (www.kleankanteen.com). Also, adding a pinch of sea salt to your water can help your body absorb the water better and reduce the frequency of needing to urinate.

Lastly, we also drink the water on our skin, 60% of the chemicals and chlorine in water is absobed through our skin. It is importmant to use filtration systems in the bath and shower, either by placing it directly on the pipe or purchasing a household water filtration system.

An excellent resource on why we need to drink water is "Your Body's Many Cries for Water" by F. Batmanghelidj, M.D.[5]

# Alcohol

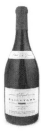

Some sources say it is ok to drink small quantities of alcohol, but "Your Pregnancy Week by Week"[10] (and other sources) recommend that no alcohol be consumed during pregnancy, as it can cause fetal alcohol syndrome (FAS). FAS occurs when alcohol crosses the placental barrier and it can stunt fetal growth or weight, create distinctive facial stigmata, damage neurons and brain structures, and cause other physical, mental, or behavioral problems. The alcohol you ingest goes directly to the baby, so by the time you are "buzzed" your baby is ready to pass out from too much alcohol. If your cravings are high, try a virgin drink, such as a virgin bloody mary or non-alcoholic beer.

# Caffeine

Caffeine is a diuretic and stimulant that gets a great deal of poor publicity, yet in most large cities, we have a coffee shop on every corner. Coffee shops are a "feel good" place to work, visit, meet and simply just hangout. For some, coffee is a necessity to start the day, while for others it gives them the jitters just smelling it. Coffee has been shown to rob our adrenal glands and deplete our hormones, as well as provide much needed antioxidants in our body.

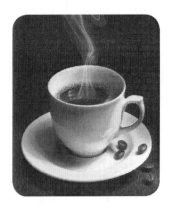

I am a coffee addict. I love the taste, the mild buzz and I have learned to drink it in moderation and have gone to great lengths to heal my body of possible damages the coffee has caused, long before pregnancy. When I found out I was pregnant, I quit drinking coffee all together. I dealt with the headaches and tiredness and once in a while I drank organic decaffeinated Swiss water processed coffee (Swiss water processed means no chemicals are used to decaffeinate the coffee). I read books that said 5 shots of espresso a day were fine for a pregnant women and I read studies that showed no amount of coffee was ok, as it could have significant effects on the brain development of my baby. Below are some recommendations from the March of Dimes[15] to help you make the best decision for you and your baby, but when in doubt, rule it out.

According to Baby Center, The March of Dimes[15] advises women to limit their caffeine intake to less than 200 mg. per day (that's about one 12-ounce cup of coffee). This recommendation was prompted by the results of a study published in the March 2008 issue of the American Journal of Obstetrics and Gynecology[2] that showed that moms-to-be who consumed 200 mg or more of caffeine a day had double the risk of miscarriage, compared with those who had no caffeine.

Not all studies show a link between caffeine consumption and a higher risk of miscarriage. Still, it may be smart to err on the side of caution and stick to the March of Dimes recommendation. (See the chart below to get a sense of the caffeine content of various types of coffee, tea, and other common sources).

Of course, if you decide to cut out caffeine altogether, you won't get any arguments from your doctor or midwife.

| Source | Mg. of Caffeine |
| --- | --- |
| Brewed Coffee - 8 oz. | 137 mg. |
| Instant Coffee - 8 oz. | 76 mg. |
| Brewed Tea - 8 oz. | 48 mg. |
| Instant Tea - 8 oz. | 26-36 mg. |
| Soft Drinks (such as cola) - 12 oz. | 37 mg. |
| Hot Cocoa (3 tsp. or 1 envelope) | 8-12 mg. |
| Chocolate Milk - 8 oz. | 5-8 mg. |
| Dark Chocolate 1.45 oz. bar | 30 mg. |
| Milk Chocolate - 1.55 oz. bar | 11 mg. |
| Chocolate Syrup - 2 tbsp. | 3 mg. |
| Coffee Ice Cream/Frozen Yogurt - 4 oz. | 2 mg. |
| Table 3: Caffeine Content In Food and Drink | |

## Are there other risks besides miscarriage?

Yes. Because caffeine causes blood vessels to constrict, it may reduce blood flow to the placenta. Caffeine easily crosses the placenta and reaches your baby (who then metabolizes it very slowly), so caffeine may directly affect your baby's developing cells.

**A study in Denmark found that the risk of stillbirth more than doubled in women who drank a great deal of coffee per day – eight cups or more – compared with women who didn't drink coffee. Some studies suggest that high caffeine consumption may slightly reduce a baby's birth weight, but other research has shown no association.[15]**

## Alternatives to coffee that are low in caffeine:

- Yerba mate
- Organic decaffeinated coffee in moderation (do not use commercial decaf coffee as it contains too many chemicals).

## Alternatives to coffee that are caffeine free:

- Herbal teas
- Pregnancy Tea by Traditional Medicinals

# A look at essential vitamins and minerals

### VITAMIN A

An excellent article on vitamins and pregnancy can be found at http://www.westonaprice.org/childrens-health/vitamins-for-fetal-development-conception-to-birth#clo[20]

Diets of healthy traditional people contain 10 times the amounts of vitamin A than the American diet. "Vitamin A is one of the several fat-soluble activators present only in animal fats and necessary for the assimilation of minerals in the diets"[20]. Foods, such as spring butter, fish eggs and liver are exceptionally rich in vitamin A. Many cultures also used liver for various types of blindness due to its high levels of vitamin A. Weston A. Price discovered that cod liver oil was even more effective than liver in restoring visual function. At the end of the First World War, a physician named Bloch discovered that a diet containing whole milk, butter, eggs and cod liver oil, cured night blindness. In one important experiment, Bloch compared the results when he fed one group of children whole milk and the other margarine as the only fat. Half of the margarine-fed children developed corneal problems while the children receiving butterfat and cod liver oil remained healthy[20].

There are many studies showing that vitamin A from animal fat sources promotes health, growth and can prevent cancer. The important thing you must remember is that getting vitamin A from fruits and vegetables (carotenes) is not the same as obtaining vitamin A from animal fat (retinol). Under optimal conditions humans can convert carotene to retinol, but it takes an awful lot of fruits and vegetables to obtain even the daily minimum requirements of vitamin A, assuming the conversion is optimal. The best sources for vitamin A are butter, egg yolk, liver, organ meats and shellfish. Beware of foods claiming to have high levels of vitamin A that is manufactured, as it is less effective than vitamin A from it's retinol source (animal fat). A few manufacturers, who are very guilty of this are, Kellogg, Cargill, Monsanto and Procter & Gamble. They have added "vitamin A" from it's carotene source to margarine, vegetable oil, wheat flour sugar and breakfast cereal – even MSG[20]. Now people all over the world believe that they are getting the vitamin A their body needs from highly processed junk food. Not true!

How much to take? The RDA (recommended daily allowance) for vitamin A is 2500 IU and has set upper limits of 10,000 IUs for women[20]. Weston A. Price recommends at least 15,000 IUs to 40,000 IUs of vitamin A a day. The anti-vitamin-A campaign began with a flawed study in 1995 from the Boston University School of Medicine. The study claimed that there was a link to high doses of vitamin A and birth defects. However, they failed to cite that most of the birth defects could also be caused by low levels of vitamin A and the study only used questionnaires to determine the levels of vitamin A mothers took and did not indicate the source of the vitamin A.

For more information on this study visit www.westonaprice.org/basicnutrition/vitaminasaga.html.[20]

When I was pregnant, I was getting a lot of headaches and began eating 3 eggs a day and 12 shrimp a day. My headaches went away and I felt healthier than ever. Eating foods rich in vitamin A, always causes a red flag to go up for most people due to the media toting it's flag that high cholesterol foods are bad. Our body needs cholesterol to produce hormones and protect joints. When you are pregnant and breastfeeding, your cholesterol will be higher than average due to the baby's need for cholesterol.

Keep in mind that when your blood cholesterol is higher than what your doctor recommends, it may actually be fine. So remember, a high-fat diet rich in vitamin A will result in steady even growth, a healthy physique and high immunity to illness for pregnant women, babies and even dads. For more information on the research cited in this section, go to www.westonaprice.org/basicnutrition/vitamindmiracle.html.

## VITAMIN D

Another extremely important fat soluble vitamin is vitamin D. Vitamin D helps prevents rickets in children, as well as promotes a high immunity to tooth decay, and resistance to disease. Furthermore, vitamin D has been found to protect against both Type I and Type II diabetes, correct Polycystic Ovarian Syndrome, increase fertility, reduce menstrual migraines and much much more.[20]

Many people think we can get the vitamin D we need from sunlight, but research shows that this may not be the case. "Humans do indeed manufacture vitamin D from cholesterol by the action of sunlight on the skin but it is actually very difficult to obtain even a minimal amount of vitamin D with a brief foray into the sunlight"[20]. The sunlight must come specifically from UV-B sunlight, which is most available from 10am – 2pm, and 85% of the body surface needs to be exposed.[20]

The best source of vitamin D is from food, such as organ meats, skin and fat from certain land animals (organic), as well as shellfish, egg yolks and oily fish. Because most of these foods are unacceptable for most people to eat due to misinformation or taste, vitamin D supplements such as high grade cod liver oil (check the source and make sure it is arsenic free) are essential. In order for vitamin D to be efficient, it is important to take it with a calcium and magnesium supplements. Vitamin D promotes calcium absorption, so without calcium present in the diet, it will be drawn from the bones.

Dr. Reinhold Vieth proved through research that the optimal amount of vitamin D we need to be vibrant and healthy is 4,000 IU compared to the 200-400 IU recommended by the RDA. Individuals with sarcoidosis, liver or kidney disease should consult their physician before supplementing with vitamin D. [20]

## FISH OILS

It is so important to take fish oils containing vitamin A, vitamin D and omega 3s. Especially for vegetarian moms. Remember if you are taking a calcium supplement, it is important to take vitamin D as well and vice versa. Westin A. Price lists some good sources for fish oils, for a complete list worldwide go to http://www.westonaprice.org/cod-liver-oil/cod-liver-oil-basics#brands.[20]

### In the United States
### BEST (Available Online/Mail Order):

- Green Pasture Products: Blue Ice High-Vitamin Fermented Cod Liver Oil  - greenpasture.org
- Dr. Ron's Ultra-Pure: Blue Ice High-Vitamin Fermented Cod Liver Oil - drrons.com
- Radiant Life: Blue Ice High-Vitamin Fermented Cod Liver Oil - 4radiantlife.com
- Natural Health Advocates: Blue Ice High-Vitamin Fermented Cod Liver Oil - building-health.com/

### GOOD (Available in Stores):

- Carlson soft gel Cod Liver Oil Super 1,000 mg capsules
- NOW double strength Cod Liver Oil capsules
- Sonne's Cod Liver Oil
- Swanson double strength Cod Liver Oil capsules
- Twin Labs non-emulsified liquid Cod Liver Oil

# Supplements

Supplementing your diet can be extremely important, even if you eat all the right foods. When you are pregnant, your baby relies so much on the nutrients you are providing him or her, and in order for that baby to thrive, you want to make sure you are getting everything you need. Many nutrients can be found in food, however the food must be from a good source, such as local growers who do not use pesticides, or organic foods. Eating foods high in folate and iron can help a great deal as well.

## Foods high in folate:

Folate is suggested as a supplement for pregnant women to take in order to prevent neural tube defects (when the neural tube in the spine and brain does not close properly) in newborn babies. Taking a folate supplement has been shown to promote tissue growth in the fetus as well as help cells to work properly. Excellent sources of folate include romaine lettuce, spinach, asparagus, turnip greens, mustard greens, calf's liver, parsley, collard greens, broccoli, cauliflower, beets, and lentils.

Very good sources include squash, black beans, pinto beans, garbanzo beans, oranges, papaya and string beans.

You need at least 600 - 1,000 mcg. of folic acid a day during your pregnancy and while you are breastfeeding. In order to get that amount through food, you need to eat 3-6 cups of the foods listed above, per day, depending on the food.

- Beans and liver are higher in folic acid than fruits and some vegetables.
- Beans average 156-357 mcg. per cup
- Vegetables average 262 mcg. per cup
- Fruit average 115 mcg. per cup
- Liver averages 860 mcg. per 4 ounces

## Foods high in iron:

Iron is essential during pregnancy because you have 50% more blood, so you need more iron to make hemoglobin (protein in red blood cells that carries oxygen). Excellent food sources of iron include chard, spinach, thyme, and turmeric. Very good sources of iron include romaine lettuce, blackstrap molasses, mustard greens, turnip greens, string beans, and shiitake mushrooms.

Good sources of iron include beef tenderloin, lentils, brussels sprouts, asparagus, venison, garbanzo beans, broccoli, leeks, and kelp.

According to the March of Dimes[15] on average you need 27 milligrams daily of iron during your pregnancy.

## Foods that provide .5 to 1.5 milligrams of iron:

- Chicken, 3 ounces
- Green peas, 1/2 cup
- Tomato juice, 6 ounces
- Broccoli, 1/2 cup
- Brussels sprouts, 1/2 cup cooked
- Whole wheat bread, 1 slice
- Dried apricots, 5 halves
- Raspberries, 1 cup
- Strawberries, 1 cup

## Foods that provide 1.6 to 3 milligrams of iron:

- Sirloin steak, 3 ounces
- Roast beef, 3 ounces
- Lean hamburger, 3 ounces
- Baked potato with skin
- Kidney beans, 1/2 cup cooked
- Lima beans, 1/2 cup cooked
- Navy beans, 1/2 cup cooked
- Oatmeal, 1 cup cooked
- Raisins, 1/2 cup

## Foods that provide 3 to 12 milligrams of iron:

- Clams, 4 large or 9 small
- Oysters, 6 medium
- Spinach, 1/2 cup cooked

## PRENATAL VITAMINS

A good prenatal vitamin is essential. Prenatal vitamins are different than the average multivitamin as they contain iron and folic acid. Please note the extra iron in a prenatal vitamin can irritate the stomach in the first trimester. Check with your doctor, as you may want to wait and take a prenatal vitamin with iron after the first trimester. Whichever brand of supplement you decide to take, make sure it is derived from an organic plant source and not synthesized.

## Good Prenatal Vitamin Sources:

- New Chapter (has traces of organic soy flour and fermented soy. Dr. Daniels mentions that fermented soy is a better choice, however, if you are concerned about soy you may want to avoid this supplement)
- Designs for Health
- Ultra life
- Dr. Schulze (www.herbdoc.com)
- Young Living (http://.holli.vibrantscents.com)

In summary, take a good prenatal vitamin and cod liver oil supplement each day, even if you feel you are eating all the right foods. Many foods today are not as nutrient rich as they should be due to poor food sources and over processing.

Lastly, Traditional Medicinals makes a tea called "pregnancy tea" that supports a healthy pregnancy.

# Eating Vegetarian When You Are Pregnant

There are many reasons people become vegetarians or vegans. This chapter is not about why. It is about how to be a "healthy" vegetarian during your pregnancy and while breastfeeding. I also encourage you to research if being a vegetarian the right choice for the health and development of your baby. Many vegetarians eat meat during their pregnancy to increase the amount of nutrients needed for fetal development. I have found four excellent references which I used to provide the best information I could on being a healthy vegetarian; *The Whole Soy Story* by Dr. Kaayla Daniels[8], www.westonaprice.org[19], www.savvyvegetarian.com[21] and HHP Coryn Leaman[13].

If you choose to remain a vegetarian during your pregnancy, it is extremely important you pay close attention to your diet to insure that you are getting enough fat and protein to help your baby grow.

### Hypospadias

is a birth defect of the urethra, in the male, that involves an abnormally placed urinary meatus (the opening, or male external urethral orifice). Instead of opening at the tip of the glans of the penis, a hypospadic urethra opens anywhere along a line (the urethral groove) running from the tip along the underside (ventral aspect) of the shaft to the junction of the penis and scrotum or perineum. A distal hypospadias may be suspected, even in an uncircumcised boy, from an abnormally formed foreskin and downward tilt of the glans.[8]

Protein is essential for optimal health and growth and it can be difficult to obtain in a vegetarian diet if you are not paying attention to the source of your foods. Be sure to combine foods properly or eat the right foods so that your body is getting the protein it needs for your baby's development. There are numerous websites available to help you decide which diet is right for you. The main thing to remember is that you are getting all the nutrients you need from your food and some from your supplements (see supplements chapter on page 207). Vegetarians tend to get little iron, B12 and Omega 3 fatty acids, as well as vitamin D and vitamin A. Further, many vegetarian diets include a great deal of soy from soy milk to soy cheese and soy hamburgers. Remember, too much soy can be damaging to your body and your baby because of increased hormones, MSG and nitrites being ingested. Soy has been found to cause *Hypospadias* in male babies when ingested by their mother's during pregnancy. Due to the high levels of phytoestrogens in soy; it has been linked to today's epidemic of infertility. Further studies have linked learning disorders, attention deficit and other behavioral disorders to infants who were fed soy formula.

I encourage you to minimize your soy intake so you are not eating soy every day, or even at all. On the next page is a quick reference to the dangers of soy and a list of soy foods that are safe to eat. *The Whole Soy Story* by Dr. Kaayla Daniel[8] is an excellent resource for further information. In addition, please reference the children's health section in *Postpartum Health and Happiness*, for information on infants and soy formula.

## Confused About Soy? - Soy Dangers Summarized

Reference: Soy Alert! www.westonaprice.org[20]

- High levels of phytic acid in soy reduce assimilation of calcium, magnesium, copper, iron and zinc. Phytic acid in soy is not neutralized by ordinary preparation methods such as soaking, sprouting and long, slow cooking. High phytate diets have caused growth problems in children.

- Trypsin inhibitors in soy interfere with protein digestion and may cause pancreatic disorders. In test animals, soy containing trypsin inhibitors caused stunted growth.

- Soy phytoestrogens disrupt endocrine function and have the potential to cause infertility and to promote breast cancer in adult women.

- Soy phytoestrogens are potent antithyroid agents that cause hypothyroidism and may cause thyroid cancer. In infants, consumption of soy formula has been linked to autoimmune thyroid disease.

- Vitamin B12 analogs in soy are not absorbed and actually increase the body's requirement for B12.

- Soy foods increase the body's requirement for vitamin D.

- Fragile proteins are denatured during high temperature processing to make soy protein isolate and textured vegetable protein.

- Processing of soy protein results in the formation of toxic lysinoalanine and highly carcinogenic nitrosamines.

- Free glutamic acid or MSG, a potent neurotoxin, is formed during soy food processing and additional amounts are added to many soy foods.

- Soy foods contain high levels of aluminum, which is toxic to the nervous system and the kidneys.

### What soy is safe to consume? by Dr. Kaayla Daniel, author of *The Whole Soy Story*

This excerpt came directly from Dr. Kaayla Daniels[8]:

"I share your concerns about GM soybeans and have covered that issue in my book. I also share your concerns about soybean processing, including matters of glutamate toxicity, and cover that issue in my book as well. My book has been endorsed by Dr. Russell Blaylock, a leading researcher on excitotoxins. In terms of safe soy consumption for those who are not allergic or sensitive to soy, I recommend small amounts of the fermented products miso, natto, tempeh, shoyu and tamari made with organic soybeans if eaten in small quantities and no more than a few times a week. That is also the position of the Weston A. Price Foundation as stated in many of its publications. I also don't worry about the occasional vegetarian potluck with tofu or whatever. But these are very hazardous for people who react poorly to MSG. However, the bottom line is that all soybeans, including organic soybeans, contain naturally occurring antinutrients, toxins and phytoestrogens that have been linked to thyroid damage, reproductive problems, infertility, ADD/ADHD, cognitive decline and a host of other problems, including heart disease and cancer growth. Although old-fashioned fermentation processes eliminate most of the antinutrients (protease inhibitors, phytates, etc.), all soybeans and soy products sold in the marketplace contain the dangerous phytoestrogens. I document this thoroughly in my book, which is 457 pages with 44 pages of references (should you wish to do your own follow up). Several chapters from my book are posted on www.westonaprice.org (The Promotion of Soy, Soy Lecithin, Soy Carbohydrates, Not Milk and Uncheese). Two Special Reports taken from the book can also be obtained free from my website."[8]

# Eating a Healthy Vegetarian Diet

I have researched some great tips on eating a healthy vegetarian diet so that you and your baby are getting the nutrients you need for a healthy pregnancy.

### Best Grain Preparation:

- Grains, nuts and seeds should either be sprouted, soaked in an acidic medium (such as lemon juice), fermented or sour-leavened in order to make them more digestible and nourishing. (Many people who are allergic to grains can tolerate them when they are prepared in this way).

### Preserving Foods:

- Consider lacto-fermentation, a method of food preservation which was used before refrigeration or canning. It is extremely easy to do and it does not involve using boiling water or heat of any kind. In this way, food enzymes are preserved, and there is actually an increase in enzyme content and vitamin content. Just about any vegetable or fruit may be naturally preserved in this way. For directions go to http://www.nourishingdays.com/2009/07/the-benefits-of-fermented-food.

### Dairy Considerations:

- The health problems which are frequently attributed to consuming dairy products are a result of over-processing and improper treatment of dairy animals--grain feeding, synthetic growth hormones, animal parts in the feed, etc. etc. Raw dairy products from healthy, exclusively grass-fed animals are very high in nutrients and these nutrients are much more available to the human body. If you are skeptical about consuming raw milk during pregnancy, or do not have access to it in your area be sure to drink organic milk. If you suspect you have dairy allergies, please read the dairy section on page 195.

Another great source that I found in my research for eating as a vegetarian is www.savvyvegetarian.com[21]. I have given an overview of the information they offer on their website, through research done by several physicians and professors in the field of nutrition.

## A Review of Protein & Essential Amino Acids From a Vegetarian Perspective

Protein is essential for health, along with carbohydrates and fats. We use protein to make building blocks, called amino acids, for every part of our bodies: blood, skin, cartilage, muscles and bones, hormones and enzymes. Our bodies can synthesize 16 of the 23 amino acids that we need. That leaves 8 essential amino acids (9 for children), which must come from the foods we eat.[21]

## The 8 Essential Amino Acids Have Important Functions In The Body:

- Isoleucine (Ile) - for muscle production, maintenance and recovery after workout. Involved in hemoglobin formation, blood sugar levels, blood clot formation and energy.

- Leucine (Leu) - growth hormone production, tissue production and repair, prevents muscle wasting, used in treating conditions such as Parkinson's disease.

- Lysine (Lys) - calcium absorption, bone development, nitrogen maintenance, tissue repair, hormone production, antibody production.

- Methionine (Met) - fat emulsification, digestion, antioxidant (cancer prevention), arterial plaque prevention (heart health), and heavy metal removal.

- Phenylalanine (Phe) - tyrosine synthesis and the neurochemicals dopamine and norepinephrine. Supports learning and memory, brain processes and mood elevation.

- Threonine (Thr) monitors bodily proteins for maintaining or recycling processes.

- Tryptophan (Trp) - niacin production, serotonin production, pain management, sleep and mood regulation.

- Valine (Val) helps muscle production, recovery, energy, endurance; balances nitrogen levels; used in treatment of alcohol related brain damage.

- Histidine (His) - the 'growth amino' essential for young children. Lack of histidine is associated with impaired speech and growth. Abundant in spirulina, seaweed, sesame, soy, rice and legumes.

## Complete and Incomplete Protein:

ALL plant based foods have varying amounts of protein (plus carbohydrates, fats and other good things), and the body will combine proteins from all sources, to make 'complete protein'. That's true for everybody, veg or non-veg. The term 'complete protein' means that all eight essential amino acids are present in the correct proportion. Foods from animal sources have complete proteins. Some foods from the plant kingdom, such as soy and quinoa, have complete protein. The term 'incomplete protein' refers to foods which have all the essential amino acids, but are low in one or more of them. That's called the 'limiting amino acid'. Most plant foods have one or more limiting amino acids, which limit the availability of all the other amino acids in the food. That's why these foods are called 'incomplete proteins'. For example, the limiting amino acid in grains is usually lysine (Lys); in legumes it can be methionine (Met) and tryptophan (Trp). So, the low level of Lys in grains is complemented by a higher level in legumes, and vice versa, to make 'complete protein'.[21]

However, vegetarians and vegans don't need to worry about complete and incomplete protein. It is NOT NECESSARY for vegetarians and vegans to combine specific protein foods at one sitting to make complete protein.[13,21]

## What Vegetarians Should Eat To Get Enough Protein

Each plant food has its own unique amino acid profile, from green leafy veggies to tubers, from barley to quinoa, from lentils to tofu, from macadamia to brazil nuts. By eating a variety of plant foods with 'incomplete proteins' throughout the day, we can easily get enough 'complete protein.' For lacto and ovo-lacto vegetarians, any food can be complemented by the high quality proteins in dairy products or eggs, but it isn't at all necessary to include animal foods to get enough protein in your diet.

Your body puts together amino acids from plant foods to give you complete protein throughout the day. For instance, the amino acids in beans & lentils are balanced by those in grains, nuts and seeds, and vice versa. Vegetables and fruits also contribute significant amounts of protein. A one cup serving of avocado, for example, has 3 grams of protein, and a medium potato with skin has 4 grams.

Vegans and vegetarians can get all the essential amino acids, by eating different combinations of grains, legumes, nuts & seeds, vegetables & fruit several times throughout the day.

Eating for complete protein isn't a scientific system of food combining, where you have to keep track and analyze everything you eat. It's a natural traditional way of eating, which most human beings have thrived on, for thousands of years. Food is a sensual pleasure, and complete protein is a side benefit.

As a rough guide, the chart below shows some examples of foods that go together well. This table is very limited. In reality, the possibilities could fill several pages, and you don't need to rely on precise combinations of food for complete protein. [21]

| Food | Limiting Amino Acids (low levels not completely missing) | Complementary Foods | Menu Item Examples |
|---|---|---|---|
| Legumes: Lentils, Peas and Beans | Tryptophan, Methionine | Grains, Nuts and Seeds | Stir-fry with green vegetables, brown rice, or Hummus with whole wheat sprouted pita bread |
| Grains: Wheat, Corn, Rice, Oats, Barley, Rye | Lysine, Isoleucine, Threonine | Legumes and Dairy | Grilled cheddar on sprouted grain bread or corn bread, chili beans and cheese |
| Nuts and Seeds: Almonds, Peanuts, Sunflower, Cashews | Lysine, Isoleucine | Legumes | Lentil walnut loaf and cashew gravy |
| Table 4: Sample vegetarian menu adapted from www.savvyvegetarian.com[21] | | | |

Author Dr. Linda Posch MS SLP ND, is a natural health care consultant, who helps her patients to achieve a healthy body balance through proper nutrition. She holds degrees in organic chemistry, psychology and a Masters in Communication Sciences and Disorders. Dr. Posch's professional background includes acute care & senior neuro-rehab, special education, autism support & therapy, spinal cord injuries, and oncology family support services.[21]

An Excellent book that offers great vegetarian recipes is:

*Forks over Knives* by Gene Stone

**www.forksoverknives.com**

---

## QUIZ #5

1.  Which fat sources are good sources for our bodies?

    _____

2.  Which foods are rich in vitamin D?

    _____

3.  What are the 2 sources of vitamin A?

    _____, _____

4.  Which 2 ingredients are known to cause digestive issues?

    _____, _____

5.  Which harmful substance is soy usually converted to during processing?

    _____

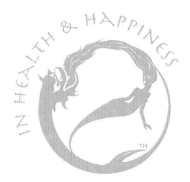

# POSTPARTUM

Postpartum Health and Happiness was developed to continue on the prenatal exercise, yoga and nutrition sections, to help you get your body back in shape. In addition, it offers mothers some helpful tips on successful breastfeeding and care of their new born baby, including what to feed them and research I have done on SIDs, mastasis, homeopathic remedies and vaccinations.

The following pages offer a glimpse of *Postpartum Health and Happiness*.

# Postpartum Exercises

For in-depth information on postpartum see *Postpartum Health and Happiness*.

Giving Birth is letting go….. Elizabeth Noble[18]

Relaxation, postpartum, is essential to the healing process. It will take your uterus 6 weeks to shrink and you will begin feeling all sorts of profound changes in your life. You may have after pains as the uterus shrinks and may not feel motivated to exercise. After I gave birth I was depressed about being overweight and anxious and stressed about losing the weight. One of my clients at the time told me – "Hang in there, after 6 months all the weight will start to come off." Now this may not be true for everyone, but if you take it easy and learn to relax, walk and enjoy your new baby, the weight will most likely come off. It did for me and several of my clients who walked, did yoga and light strength training exercises. Exercise is stress and if you are doing stressful exercises during a time of high stress in your life, the exercise becomes a road block to losing weight, not a tool for losing weight.

The best way to begin getting back into shape after the baby, is walking. Walking helps you get out of the house with your baby and slowly introduces your body to exercise again. Giving birth can be very hard on the body and it can take up to 2 years for the body to completely heal. Take it easy the first 6 months and focus on exercises that make you feel good and restore strength and stability to your body and your mind.

## After A Vaginal Birth

Most likely you will be able to exercise within a week after giving birth. If you have stitches, make sure the exercise is light and there is little pain or discomfort during exercise. Sitz baths are essential, so consider using a herbal tea sitz bath such as Motherlove Herbal Company Sitz Bath Concentrate. The combination of witch hazel leaf, yarrow, uva ursi, grain alcohol, and distilled water is a great way to sooth yourself after birth. The combination of herbs also soothes sore perineal muscles, reduces swelling, slows bleeding, and heals tears.

## After A Cesarean Birth

If you had a C-section and you were committed to natural child birth, it is often a huge disappointment and you may have feelings of inadequacy and self doubt. For those of us who had a c-section when all you wanted was a natural child birth, there are support groups out there that can be found on http://community.babycenter.com/groups[4].

It is important to start moving as soon as possible. Performing easy breathing exercises to help clear your body of the effects of the anesthetics are essential. Light walking is extremely important. You will most likely be on pain medication post surgery, but remember that pain is your guide to help determine when you are doing too much. After my c-section I was told that I could not walk up stairs and had to rest as much as possible and must take my pain medication. Are you kidding me? I did not take my pain medication after the 2nd day out of the hospital, I had to walk up stairs in my home and I had a baby and 2 dogs to take care of. I listened to my body and when my scar hurt, I backed off for a few hours and took it easy. I was walking my dogs 10 minutes a day and taking stairs, but I was always mindful of my scar hurting.

Within 6 weeks after your C-section (or when your physician gives you the clearance to do so), start to massage the c-section scar a few minutes every day with organic helichrysum or rose hip oil. Techniques for massage can be found on Youtube.com or ask your massage therapist to show you how. This will break down the scar tissue the body develops, which can cause problems by binding together body parts that are normally unconnected. Rose hip oil improves surgical and accidental scars, and avoids the formation of the keloid type of scar, (lump) which may appear after surgical procedures. Massaging your c-section scar can also help avoid incontinence, as well as reduce pain. Massaging your scar helps it to heal faster because it increases circulation and connection, stimulating the healing process.

You will need time for emotional healing after a c-section, so get help if you need to talk to someone. Most insurance plans cover psychologists visits for postpartum women, so do take advantage of it.

# Breastfeeding

According to my research, breastfeeding is the best choice for you and your baby if it is something your body and your lifestyle allows you to do. In fact, breastfeeding has become so important to the health and well being for both babies and mothers, that the American Academy of Pediatrics[1] came out with the following statement on-line on February 27, 2012:

> *Breastfeeding and human milk are the normative standards for infant feeding and nutrition. Given the documented short- and long-term medical and neurodevelopmental advantages of breastfeeding, infant nutrition should be considered a public health issue and not only a lifestyle choice. The American Academy of Pediatrics reaffirms its recommendation of exclusive breastfeeding for about 6 months, followed by continued breastfeeding as complementary foods are introduced, with continuation of breastfeeding for 1 year or longer as mutually desired by mother and infant. Medical contraindications to breastfeeding are rare. Infant growth should be monitored with the World Health Organization (WHO) Growth Curve Standards to avoid mislabeling infants as underweight or failing to thrive. Hospital routines to encourage and support the initiation and sustaining of exclusive breastfeeding should be based on the American Academy of Pediatrics-endorsed WHO/UNICEF "Ten Steps to Successful Breastfeeding." National strategies supported by the US Surgeon General's Call to Action, the Centers for Disease Control and Prevention, and The Joint Commission are involved to facilitate breastfeeding practices in US hospitals and communities. Pediatricians play a critical role in their practices and communities as advocates of breastfeeding and thus should be knowledgeable about the health risks of not breastfeeding, the economic benefits to society of breastfeeding, and the techniques for managing and supporting the breastfeeding dyad. The "Business Case for Breastfeeding" details how mothers can maintain lactation in the workplace and the benefits to employers who facilitate this practice.*
>
> For more information go to www.aap.org/

**Further, The Center for Disease control made the following commitment:**
CDC's Division of Nutrition, Physical Activity, and Obesity (DNPAO) is committed to increasing breastfeeding rates throughout the United States and to promoting and supporting optimal breastfeeding practices toward the ultimate goal of improving the public's health.

Breastfeeding may not fit into everyone's lifestyle and not everyone can breast feed, but if you choose not to breast feed for lifestyle reasons, it is important that you understand the benefits of breastfeeding before you decide to bottle feed. Woman who must to return to work can still give their babies a healthy start, even if they cannot breast feed longer than a month. Further, make sure you attend a breastfeeding support group prior to giving birth to help answer as many questions as possible. Once your baby is born, you will be sleep deprived and unable to do the research you need to should you have problems breastfeeding. For more information on breastfeeding, please see Postpartum Health and Happiness.

## A great way to find breastfeeding support groups and information on all your breastfeeding questions prior to giving birth can be found on the following websites:

http://www.breastfeeding.org
http://www.llli.org/ La Leche League International
http://lllusa.org/La Leche League USA
http://babyfriendlyusa.org/
www.americanpregnancy.org
www.womenshealth.gov
www.westonaprice.org
www.aap.org

# Mastitis

Mastitis occurs infrequently, but can be quite painful and usually occurs between the 10th and 28th day postpartum. When a breast infection does occur, it is important for the mother to seek prompt medical attention from her primary care provider. This will lead to a speedy resolution and avoid further complications. In addition, a mother needs to know that she can safely continue to breast feed.[1,15]

## SIGNS

Women with a breast infection (mastitis) often describe flu-like symptoms, including weakness, headache, nausea, soreness, chills, and fever (greater than 101 degrees F or 38.4 degrees C). The breast can be red, hot, and painful.[15]

## CAUSES

When breastfeedings are infrequent, the breasts are not emptied completely, missed, or when babies are positioned incorrectly on the breast, milk collects in the breast and puts pressure on surrounding tissue, causing engorgement. Engorgement damages the tissue and increases the risk of infection. When bacteria enter the breast through an opening in the nipple or a break in the skin, the damaged tissue becomes infected.

## RECOMMENDED TREATMENT

- Call your doctor. An antibiotic may be necessary. Take the antibiotic until it is gone, even if your symptoms improve.
- Put warm water on the infected area before each breastfeeding to aid let-down and relieve pain. Warm washcloths, a warm shower or bath, or soaking the breasts in a pan of warm water works well.
- Continue to breast feed frequently on both breasts. Breast feed every 1-3 hours during the day and every 2-3 hours at night.
- Start each feeding on the uninfected breast until the let-down reflex occurs, then switch to the infected breast. Breast feed only until the breast is soft. If necessary, hand express or pump to soften the breast.
- Apply cold packs after each breastfeeding to relieve pain and reduce swelling. Bags of frozen peas wrapped in a cold washcloth work well.
- Place cold cabbage in your bra to relieve symptoms.
- Place frankesense oil on your palms or heels several times a day. [27]
- Drink enough fluid to satisfy your thirst. Water and unsweetened fruit juices are best.
- Get plenty of rest.

## PREVENTION

- Position the baby correctly on the breast and use 2-3 different breastfeeding positions each day.
- Do not delay or miss feedings, but if you do, or if the baby breast feeds poorly, hand express or pump to soften the breasts and relieve fullness.
- Avoid bras that are too tight or that bind and bras with under wire.
- Wean gradually. Pump or hand express to soften the breasts and relieve fullness.

# Postpartum Depression

Entering the world of motherhood changes us in so many ways, both positive and negative. Many woman have severe postpartum blues and contemplate hurting themselves and even their children. Our hormones are out of balance, our lives are out of balance, we can feel isolated and alone. As women we strive to "DO IT ALL" ourselves. We live in a time of women being independent, self reliant and too proud or too scared to ask for help.

Help is out there and is not a luxury, but a necessity. In most countries woman have a midwife help them for at least the first 15 days after their baby is born, some countries 1-3 months. Women need to heal after birth and the healing process cannot take place unless someone is there to help with your newborn baby.

Start building a network for yourself of people than can help you and connect with you once your baby is born. Ask family and friends for help, find a community of support through organizations liked sacred pregnancy. Hiring a Doula is a great way to go as well, as they not only help you with your baby, but can answer your questions and help with breastfeeding issues. Talk to your doctor about counseling and support systems they may know about through the hospital. Below are some resources for you to begin creating a circle of friends and a circle of nurturing and loving friends.

## RESOURCES

www.sacredpregnancy.com

www.acog.org

www.dona.org (Doula's)

www.doulas.com

www.babycenter.com

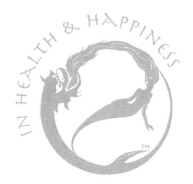

# SUMMARY

# Summary

There are so many books out there these days and everyone has an opinion about the care of your baby. What I found worked best for me, was to take in as much as I could and make my decisions by discussing everything with my partner or another parent. I often felt paralyzed about some decisions, such as vaccinations, and had to learn to just let go and do what we felt was best at the time with the information we had.

Sometimes it feels good to stop reading and just go with your gut. We live in an age of so much information that we become overwhelmed and forget that cavemen and cavewomen were parents too, and they parented with intuition and love. Enjoy your pregnancy and enjoy your baby. It does go by fast and it is important to live in the present. It is called the present because it is a gift.

# Additional Resources

## General Baby and Pregnancy Books

- The Baby Book by Dr. Sears
- Essential Exercises for the Child Bearing Years by Elizabeth Noble
- What to Expect When You're Expecting by Heidi Murkoff, Arlene Eisenberg and Sandee Hathaway, B.S.N
- Baby Wise by Gary Ezzo and Robert Bucknam
- What to Expect the First Year by Heidi Murkoff, Arlene Eisenberg and Sandee Hathaway, B.S.N
- Your Pregnancy Week by Week by Glade B. Curtis and Judith Schuler
- Hypnobirthing by Marie F. Mongan and Lorne R. Campbell
- www.babycenter.com (sign up for week by week e-mails about your pregnancy milestones and baby milestones)
- Belly Laughs: The Naked Truth About Pregnancy And Childbirth by Jenny McCarthy - an excellent book for those times when everything is crashing around you and you just need to laugh!

## Nutritional Resources

- The Whole Soy Story by Dr. Kaayla Daniels
- How to Eat Move and Be Healthy! by Paul Chek
- Your Bodies Many Cries for Water by Fereydoon Batmanghelidj
- The Metabolic Typing Diet by Dr. Wolcott - www.healthexcel.com
- www.westonaprice.org
- Nourishing Traditions by Sally Fallon
- www.savvyvegatarian.com
- Coryn Leaman - www.aohstore.com
- www.organicconsumers.org
- Forks over Knives by Gene Stone

## Supplemental Resources

- New Chapter
- Designs for Health
- Dr. Schulze - www.herbdoc.com
- Young Living - http://www.inhealthandhappiness.com/category/young-living-essential-oils/

# EQUIPMENT RESOURCES

Swiss balls  (Physioballs) - The ball size you should order is based on your height, see below. Remember, the ball is a good fit for you when you sit on the ball, your thighs are parallel to the floor or slightly higher.

Spri-Products - www.spriproducts.com
Fitter - www.fitter1.com
Duraball Pro - www.amazon.com - the best ball on the market

Up to 5'2" - 45cm ball
5'2" - 5'8" - 55cm ball
5'8" - 6'2" - 65cm ball
Over 6'2"  - 75cm ball

## Bosu Balls and Airex Pads and other unstable devices

Spri Products - www.gaiam.com/spri
Fitter - www.fitter1.com
Power Systems - www.power-systems.com
OPTP - www.optp.com

## Rubber Tubing

Spri Products - www.gaiam.com/spri
Power Systems - www.power-systems.com

## Foam Rollers

Foam rollers can be cheap and flatten out easily as well as cause allergies. OPTP sells an ETHA foam roller that does not breakdown easily and is hypo allergenic. Start with the white or silver foam roller, as it is softer and the 36x4 inch is best, as it better for mobilizing the vertebrae. OPTP - optp.com

## Blood Pressure Cuff

Stabilizer pressure biofeedback mechanism - www.optp.com (similar to blood pressure cuff, made specifically for abdominal exercises).
ADC Blood pressure cuff traditional - www.amazon.com or www.adctoday.com

## Compression Belts and Maternity Belts

Compression belt - OPTP - www.optp.com
Maternity belt - www.motherhood.com

## Kettlebells

For the uses in this manual you can purchase kettlebells at Target or a sporting good store. Online companies such as Power-Systems and Spri Products will have better kettlebells.
Power Systems - www.power-systems.com
Spri Products - www.gaiam.com/spri

# BABY SUPPLIES YOU NEED BEFORE YOUR BABY IS BORN

## Baby Swaddles and Carriers

- Ergo carrier - www.diapers.com or www.amazon.com (excellent for carrying your baby in the front and converts to a baby backpack as well. I used this until my son was 2 1/2.
- Moby Wrap - www.amazon.com
- Muslin clothes (adent and anais)- www.amazon.com

## Cloth Diapers - it really is easier than you think

**Chinese prefolds** (cotton diapers, ask your midwife how to fold them) - blueberrydiapers.com, www.greenmountaindiapers.com, www.zoolikins.com (be sure to buy the 3 prong fasteners)
**Diaper covers** - wool and plastic - www.tinybirdorganics.com, clothdiapers.com, www.zoolikins.com
**Waterproof diaper bag** - any of the above companies - I put them in a waterproof bag in a tall kitchen trash can with a lid and the smell was minimal.
**Wipes** - any of the above companies - I filled a spray bottle with lavender oil and water and used it with the cloth wipes

Washing Instructions: rinse poopy diapers in the toilet and then they can be placed in diaper bin. Wash every day or every other day. First cycle on hot with NO detergent. Second cycle, wash in hot water and use very little detergent along with BioKleen or Seventh Generation natural oxy stain remover. This will get them very clean.

# EXERCISE RESOURCES

## Group Fitness Instructors

American Council on Exercise - www.acefitness.org
IDEA - idea-fit.com

## Aqua Instructors

www.aeawave.com

## Yoga Instructors - instructors should hold a 200 hour yoga teaching certificate

www.idea-fit.com
www.yogaworks.com
www.yogaalliance.org

## Personal Trainer Resources

C.H.E.K Institute - www.chekinstitute.com
American Council on Exercise - www.acefitness.org
National Strength and Conditioning Association - www.nsca-lift.org
American College of Sports Medicine - www.acsm.org

## Yoga Books and Websites

www.yogajournal.com
Light on Yoga by B.K.S. Iyengar
Yoga Basics by Mara Carrico
www.namastacy.com

# HIRE A DOULA

Consider hiring a Doula to help you through your pregnancy and birth. I had a Doula and she was such a wonderful support for me during my pregnancy and during my sons birth. See the resources below for more information on hiring a Doula.

- www.dona.org (Doula's)
- www.doulas.com
- www.bellybelly.com

# References

1. American Academy of Pediatrics - www.aap.org

2. American Congress of Obstetricians and Gynecologists - www.acog.org

3. American Journal of Clinical Nutrition, Vol. 71, No. 1, 171S-175S, January 2000 (http://www.ajcn.org/content/71/1/171S.abstract).

4. Baby Center - www.babycenter.com

5. Batmanghelidj, Fereydoon *Your Bodies Many Cries for Water, Global Health Solutions, Inc.*; Third Edition edition (November 1, 2008) - ISBN-10: 0970245882

6. Chek, Paul. *How to Eat, Move and Be Healthy!*, C.H.E.K Institute, 2004 - ISBN-10: 1583870067

7. Cohen, Robert - www.notmilk.com

8. Daniels, Kaayla Dr., *The Whole Soy Story: The Dark Side of America's Favorite Health Food.*, Newtrends Publishing, Inc.; 1st edition (March 10, 2005) - ISBN-10: 0967089751

9. Fallon, Sally and Mary Enig. *Nourishing Traditions: The Cookbook that Challenges Politically Correct Nutrition and the Diet Dictocrats.* Newtrends Publishing, Inc.; Revised and Updated 2nd edition (October 1, 1999) - ISBN-10: 0967089735

10. Glade B., Curtis and Judith Schuler, M.S.. *Your Pregnancy Week by Week.* Da Capo Press, 1994. ISBN-10: 0738214647

11. Hyman, Mark Dr. - www.drhyman.com

12. Iyengar, B.K.S., Light on Yoga., Schocken; Revised edition (January 3, 1995) - ISBN-10: 0805210318

13. Leaman, Coryn. *The Length of Your Arm Lifestyle*, 1995 - www.aohstore.com

14. Livestrong.com

15. March of Dimes - www.marchofdimes.com

16. Murkoff, Heidi and Arlene Eisenberg and Sandee Hathaway B.S.N. *What to Expect When Your Expecting.* Workman Publishing Company Inc., NY, NY 2002. - ISBN-10: 0761148574

17. National Resources Defense Council - www.nrdc.org

18. Noble, Elizabeth. *Essential Exercises for the Child Bearing Years, A Guide to Health and Comfort Before and After Your Baby is Born,* 4th Edition. New Life Images, 1995. - ISBN-10: 0964118319

19. Organic Consumers Association - www.organicconsumers.org

20. Price, Weston A., Weston A. Price Foundation. - www.westonaprice.org

21. Savvy Vegetarian - http://www.savvyvegetarian.com/

22. Sears, William and Martha Dr., Little, Brown and Company; Revised edition (March 2003) - ISBN-10: 0316778001

23. United States Department of Agriculture - www.choosemyplate.gov

24. Wikipedia - www.wikipedia.com

25. Wolcott, Williams and Trish Fahey. *The Metabolic Typing Diet.* Three Rivers Press; 1st Bway Bks Tr Ppbk Ed 2002 edition (January 2, 2002) - ISBN-10: 0767905644

26. Yoga Journal - www.yogajournal.com

27. Young Living Essential Oils - http://www.inhealthandhappiness.com/category/young-living-essential-oils/

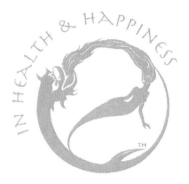

# EXAM

# How to Complete Your Exam

When you have grasped the concepts and techniques presented in this course, you are ready to take the exam.

## General Instructions

- Only one person may take this exam, receive a certificate of completion and receive continuing education credits for this exam. Please contact In Health and Happiness if you have any questions.

- This is an open book exam.

- There is only one correct answer for each question. Select the best possible answer. Choose the correct letter (A/B/C/D) for your answers to the multiple choice questions or the correct option for True/False questions (A or B).

- You must apply what you have learned from the concepts and techniques presented in this course in order to answer some of the exam questions.

## Pass Mark

The pass mark is 80%. Each question is worth 2 points. You will need to score at least 80 points of the possible 100 points.

## Retake Information

- The majority of people pass the exam the first time, as long as they have thoroughly studied the manual.

- If you do not pass the exam, you may retake it for a fee of US $25.

## To take your exam:

1. Complete the exam sheet with name, address and e-mail.

2. There is only one correct answer for each question. Select the best possible answer.

3. Choose one correct letter (A/B/C/D) for the multiple choice answers or the correct option (A/B) for True/False questions.

4. Complete the answer sheet on page 236 in the manual.

5. Keep a copy of your exam for your records, as your exam will not be returned to you.

6. Mail, e-mail or fax your Exam Answer Sheet, including registration number and Grading Request Sheet to:

In Health and Happiness
1966 Spanish Oak Way
Vista, CA 92081 USA

E-mail: holli@inhealthandhappiness.com

---

## COURSE CRITIQUE

We would appreciate your feedback and comments on this course, so we can improve this and future courses. Please take a few moments to fill in the course critique on page 237 and send it in to us with your test.

## TESTIMONIALS

We love to hear how you have benefited from this course in particular. We also use testimonials in our marketing, and offer a "thank-you" gift to anyone who provides a powerful testimonial that we use in our marketing. If you would like to share your thoughts and successes with us, please complete the Testimonial form on page 238, or send us an e-mail to holli@inhealthandhappiness.com.

# Prenatal Health and Happiness Exam

1. Which muscle(s) are key in keeping the back strong during pregnancy?

    A. Glutes and erector spinae
    B. Hamstrings and quadratus lumborum
    C. Glutes and Rectus abdominis
    D. Hamstrings and glutes

2. A Sudden stabbing pain in the groin area during pregnancy is often a result_____

    A. Tight adductors
    B. Broad ligament pain
    C. Round ligament pain
    D. Tight abductors

3. If a client has sacroiliac joint pain, which of the following exercises would be best for providing joint stability?

    A. Back extensions
    B. Abdominal crunch
    C. Alternate superman
    D. Sumo squat

4. _____ is a bacteria that causes serious infection in pregnant women and newborns.

    A. Fungus
    B. Listeria
    C. E-Coli
    D. MSG

5. What is the technical name of the abdominal wall splitting during pregnancy?

    A. Sacroiliac syndrome
    B. Round ligament strain
    C. Diastasis recti
    D. Rectus hemorrhage

6. Weak pelvic floor muscles can lead to _____.

    A. Incontinence
    B. Diastasis recti
    C. Listeria
    D. Mastitis

7. Which hormone is present in 10 times its normal concentration during pregnancy?

    A. Estrogen
    B. Progesterone
    C. Relaxin
    D. Testosterone

8. As a mother's belly and breast get bigger, which area of the body tends to become rounded?

    A. Thoracic extensors
    B. Lumbar erectors
    C. Cervical extensors
    D. Lumbar extensors

9. Wrist strength is important to develop during pregnancy.

    A. True
    B. False

10. If your core temperate exceeds _____ , you will place your baby at risk.

    A. 100 degrees
    B. 96 degrees
    C. 102 degrees
    D. 98 degrees

11. A neutral spine is when the thoracic spine is at _____ curve and the lumbar spine is at a _____ curve.

    A. 55 degree; 20 degree
    B. 35 degree; 35 degree
    C. 40 degree; 45 degree
    D. 60 degree; 25 degree

12. The right Swiss ball size for some 5'4" is:

    A. 55 cm
    B. 65 cm
    C. 75 cm
    D. 45 cm

13. Good posture allows us to handle the loads placed upon our bodies.

    A. True
    B. False

14. Forward head posture can be corrected with which exercise?

    A. Hip extension
    B. Superwoman
    C. Crawl pattern
    D. Wall lean

15. When taking a full deep breath you should breathe into the chest first.

    A. True
    B. False

16. Which exercise helps to integrate the left and right sides of the body?

    A. Crawl pattern
    B. Bent over row
    C. Sumo squat
    D. Wall push up

17. The best type of stretching for a pregnant woman would be _____.

    A. Long static holds
    B. Ballistic stretching
    C. Mobilizations
    D. No stretching

18. The best size foam roller for mobilizing the thoracic spine is:

    A. 3 feet by 4 inches
    B. 4 feet by 6 inches
    C. 3 feet by 5 inches
    D. 4 feet by 8 inches

19. A good mobilization for the pelvis is:

    A. Vertical foam roller mobilization
    B. Swiss ball hamstring stretch
    C. Groin stretch
    D. Swiss ball pelvic tilt

20. Which stretch best reduces anterior pelvic tilt?

    A. Swiss ball hamstring stretch
    B. Swiss ball hip flexor stretch
    C. Swiss ball pelvic tilt
    D. Swiss ball pec stretch

21. Spinal rotation exercises are safe for all pregnant women.

    A. True
    B. False

22. Which exercise provides excellent lifting mechanics?

    A. Sumo squat
    B. Hip extension
    C. Bent over row
    D. Swiss ball hip extension

23. During the hip extension, it is important to have your palms facing the ceiling.

    A. True
    B. False

24. When performing the toe touch drill, the knee should track over the _____.

   A. Ankle
   B. Second toe
   C. The big toe
   D. Pinky toe

25. Which exercise helps strengthen the wrists?

   A. Bent over row
   B. Crawl pattern
   C. Bench press holding dumbbells vertical
   D. Swiss ball chest fly

26. Standing on an unstable platform helps train the nervous system.

   A. True
   B. False

27. Which yoga pose helps with leg cramps?

   A. Leg elevation
   B. Forward bend
   C. Boat pose
   D. Spinal twists

28. The wide-legged forward bend helps with _____.

   A. Flat feet
   B. Headaches
   C. Quadriceps stretch
   D. Emotional release

29. Where should the tongue be placed in order to help stabilize the neck?

   A. On the bottom of the mouth
   B. It does not matter
   C. On the roof of the mouth
   D. Behind the bottom teeth

30. During standing yoga poses, the knee should be_____.

   A. In line with the ankle
   B. Behind the ankle
   C. 1 inch in front of the ankle
   D. 2 inches from the toes

31. Inversions are good for pregnant women to do.

   A. True
   B. False

32. Which pose(s) helps pump spinal fluid through the spine?

    A.    Downward dog
    B.    Cat and Cow
    C.    Seated meditation
    D.    Warrior I

33. Which pose is known to help with labor?

    A.    Cobbler's pose
    B.    Seated forward fold
    C.    Mountain pose
    D.    Standing back bend

34. Which part of our body holds emotions?

    A.    Hamstrings
    B.    Shoulders
    C.    Hips
    D.    Abdomen

35. How much water should you drink a day?

    A.    64 ounces
    B.    Eight – eight ounce glasses
    C.    Half your body weight in ounces
    D.    32 ounces

36. Nitrites are harmless in our foods.

    A.    True
    B.    False

37. Soy products usually contain MSG.

    A.    True
    B.    False

38. High fructose corn syrup can inhibit _____ metabolism.

    A.    Sodium
    B.    Magnesium
    C.    Potassium
    D.    Copper

39. A serving of fruit provides the same nutritional value whether it is in juice, a can or fresh.

    A.    True
    B.    False

40. What percent of the population is gluten intolerant?

   A. 50
   B. 20
   C. 70
   D. 60

41. Which fats are harmful to the body?

   A. Cholesterol
   B. Polyunsaturated
   C. Trans-fatty acids
   D. Monounsaturated

42. According to Weston A. Price, what is the best source of fish oil?

   A. Cod liver
   B. Salmon
   C. A mixture
   D. Krill oil

43. A good source of vitamin A can be found in most vegetables.

   A. True
   B. False

44. What helps line the gut of a new born baby?

   A. Formula
   B. Colostrums
   C. Hind milk
   D. Soy

45. Mastitis usually occurs between the _____ and _____ day postpartum.

   A. 10th and 28th
   B. 5th and 15th
   C. 15th and 30th
   D. 1st and 10th

46. The term "complete" protein means that _____.

   A. The protein source came from an animal.
   B. The food has the right combination of fats, protein and carbohydrates.
   C. The animal source was fed only grass and gluten free meal.
   D. All eight essential amino acids are present in the correct proportions.

47. The best way to prepare grains is to:

   A. Sprout them
   B. Bake them
   C. Eat them raw
   D. Boil them

48. A birth defect of the urethra in the male that involves an abnormally placed urinary meatus is called:

   A. Hyperplasia
   B. Hypospadias
   C. Diastasis
   D. Preeclampsia

49. How many milligrams of iron per day do you need during pregnancy?

   A. 30
   B. 10
   C. 50
   D. 70

50. The best source for vitamin D is:

   A. Organ meat and shellfish
   B. Whole organic milk
   C. Natural sunlight
   D. Low fat yogurt

# Answer Sheet for Prenatal Health and Happiness Exam

Name: _Amanda J. Klett_      Date: _7-1-18_
(as you would like it to appear on your certificate)

Billing Address: Apt./Ste. _7510 Highland Dr._

City: _Everett_    State: _WA_    Zip Code: _98203_

Country: _U.S.A._

E-mail: _amanda.peakeverett @ gmail.com_

Occupation: _Personal Trainer_

Phone: _425-239-6385_      Fax: _N/A_

There is only one correct answer for each question. Select the best possible answer. Choose the correct letter (A/B/C/D) for your answers to the multiple choice questions or the correct option for True/False questions (A or B). Circle the letter or place an X through it. A fill in PDF version of this exam can be found at www.inhealthandhappiness.com/resources/forms.

| | | | |
|---|---|---|---|
| 1) A B C **D** | 16) **A** B C D | 31) A **B** C D | 46) A B C **D** |
| 2) A B **C** D | 17) A B **C** D | 32) A **B** C D | 47) **A** B C D |
| 3) A B C **D** | 18) **A** B C D | 33) **A** B C D | 48) A **B** C D |
| 4) A B **C** D | 19) A B C **D** | 34) A B **C** D | 49) **A** B C D |
| 5) A B **C** D | 20) A **B** C D | 35) A B **C** D | 50) **A** B C D |
| 6) **A** B C D | 21) A **B** C D | 36) A **B** C D | |
| 7) A B **C** D | 22) **A** B C D | 37) **A** B C D | |
| 8) **A** B C D | 23) **A** B C D | 38) A B C **D** | |
| 9) **A** B C D | 24) A **B** C D | 39) **A** B C D | |
| 10) A B **C** D | 25) A B C **D** | 40) **A** B C D | |
| 11) A **B** C D | 26) **A** B C D | 41) A B **C** D | |
| 12) **A** B C D | 27) **A** B C D | 42) **A** B C D | |
| 13) **A** B C D | 28) A B C **D** | 43) A **B** C D | |
| 14) A B C **D** | 29) A B **C** D | 44) A **B** C D | |
| 15) A **B** C D | 30) **A** B C D | 45) **A** B C D | |

## Send To:

In Health and Happiness
1966 Spanish Oak Way, Vista, CA 92081
E-mail: holli@inhealthandhappiness.com

# Course Critique

Name: Amanda J. Klett      Date: _____

Occupation: Personal Trainer    Where did you purchase this course? Online

**(Please rate on scale of 1 to 5; 1 being the lowest and 5 being the highest – circle one)**

| | |
|---|---|
| Quality of materials presented | 1 2 3 ④ 5 |
| Information was academically accurate and educationally sound | 1 2 3 ④ 5 |
| Requirements for course completion were explained well | 1 2 3 4 ⑤ |
| The post-completion test was a valuable tool for measuring the amount of knowledge gained | 1 2 3 4 ⑤ |
| The level of difficulty was appropriate for my profession | 1 2 3 4 ⑤ |
| The course provided useful information for my profession | 1 2 3 4 ⑤ |
| My expectations were met | 1 2 3 4 ⑤ |

What did you like most about this course?


How would you like to see this course improve for future participants?



Would you recommend this course to a friend or professional colleague? Y/N    Why or why not?

Yes. Easy to read + understand. Received my materials in a timely manner.

What other courses or topics would interest you in the future?



Do you know anyone who would be interested in receiving information on In Health and Happiness? If you do, please list their names, addresses and/or phone numbers on the back of this page. We would be delighted to send them some information.

Thank you for your participation.

Providing this information constitutes your permission for In Health and Happiness to contact you regarding related information via mail, e-mail, fax and phone.

☐ Please check this box if you do not wish to be contacted about future events.

# Request for Testimonials

We are always appreciative of testimonials from colleagues and students that we can use to show prospective students how the programs can benefit them. Please take a moment to submit a testimonial. You can also e-mail your testimonial to holli@inhealthandhappiness.com.

Here are a few ideas to get you going:

- How has this correspondence course helped you in your profession?

- What specific skills or knowledge have you learned that have been particularly beneficial?

- Can you tell us about any particular success that you have achieved with a client?

I, (print name) _____ authorize In Health and Happiness to use the following statement(s) for promotional purposes.

_____

_____

_____

_____

_____

_____

_____

_____

Signature: _____ Date:_____

Occupation:_____